BRIDGING THE SILENCE

Understanding Patient Psychology, Misconceptions And Systemic Gaps In Indian Healthcare.

DR. ARUSHI CHANDRA

COPYRIGHT PAGE

Bridging the Silence

This is a work of nonfiction. The stories, while inspired by real events and people, have been shared with permission or anonymized to protect privacy. All health-related reflections are based on the author's personal and professional experiences and should not be taken as medical advice.

ISBN: 978-93-342-8510-9

Self-Published
Printed in India

First Edition, 2025

ABOUT THE AUTHOR

Dr. Arushi Chandra is a dentist, researcher, MBA student at IIM Indore, and storyteller whose work lies at the intersection of healthcare and humanity. A graduate of ITS - Centre for Dental Studies and Research, she has worked extensively in both clinical settings and outreach programs, with a special interest in oral health awareness and community psychology. Through her writing, she gives voice to the unheard experiences of patients and practitioners, believing that true healing begins with understanding. Bridging the Silence is her first book.

DEDICATION PAGE

For my family—my mother, my brother, and the memory of my father.
To my college, ITS - Centre for Dental Studies and Research, for shaping my roots.
To every patient who trusted me with their silence.
This is for you.

ACKNOWLEDGMENTS

This book began as a research project.
But it became something more—because of the people who stood beside me, guided me, challenged me, and trusted me even before I trusted myself.

To my Director - Principal, Dr. Devi Charan Shetty, thank you for your inspiring leadership and for building an environment where learning extended beyond textbooks—into compassion, curiosity, and care.

To the Department of Public Health Dentistry, thank you for being the foundation on which this research was built. Your constant support, guidance, and belief in this project turned a classroom idea into something deeply real and meaningful.

To the entire faculty of ITS-CDSR, thank you for shaping my skills and sensibilities. Every clinic round, every late-hour discussion, and ever real-world case added another layer to my understanding.

To my co-interns and juniors—thank you for walking this journey with me. The long hours, the shared laughter, the last-minute case discussions and chai breaks—they weren't just passing moments. They were the building blocks of who I was becoming.

To the chairside assistants, helpers, and support staff—thank you for your quiet, tireless presence. You were the heartbeat behind the scenes.

To the incredible team behind our community outreach and dental camps—thank you for showing me dentistry beyond the four walls of the clinic - one shaped by simplicity, humanity, and the power of presence. From setting up camps to seeing patients under trees or in crowded school rooms, you reminded me of why I chose this field.

To the patients—who opened not just their mouths but their stories—thank you. Your courage, your vulnerability, and your trust taught me lessons no journal ever could.

And a special thanks to Parth Bhagat—for being my unwavering source of strength. Your faith in me, your constant encouragement, and the way you always reminded me of my potential gave me the courage to dream bigger and do better. You have been my greatest supporter through every step of this journey.
This book may carry my name on its cover,

But it holds the efforts, kindness, and spirit of many.

With all my heart,
Dr. Arushi Chandra

FOREWORD

It is a rare pleasure to witness a student transform not only through academic excellence but through empathy-driven inquiry. Dr. Arushi Chandra's work, Bridging the Silence, addresses a deeply overlooked dimension of dentistry—why so many patients delay seeking care, and what we can do about it.

What begins as reflection evolves into solution. Her thoughtful integration of patient voices, behavioral insights, and practical frameworks makes this book both emotional and actionable.
It is not only a contribution to dentistry, but to public health strategy at large.

As her Director - Pricipal, I have seen her dedication first-hand. This book reflects her compassion, her clarity, and her emerging leadership in healthcare.

This book doesn't just ask questions or tell stories—it offers blueprints for change.

"Wishing Dr. Arushi all the best as she turns deep insight into impactful action. May your voice stay strong, your values stay clear, and your purpose always lead the way."

— With blessings

Dr. Devi Charan Shetty
Director - Principal
ITS - Centre For Dental Studies And Research

AUTHOR'S NOTE

This book was not written simply to recount observations—it was born out of a need to understand. Why do people delay treatment, even when they know it's necessary? Why does silence persist, even in pain? And most importantly, how can we bridge this silence?

As a dentist, I've come to appreciate that real solutions don't begin in boardrooms—they begin at the bedside. This work combines emotional insights, human psychology, and structured data to tell a story that is at once personal and systemic. My aim is to approach challenges with empathy, structure, and a drive for action.

This is more than a healthcare narrative; it is a call to rethink how we approach systems, behaviors, and change. I hope this book shows you not just who I am, but how I think.

This book begins with listening—but it ends with action. Through frameworks and cross-functional thinking, I attempt to move from insight to impact.

— Dr. Arushi Chandra

AT A GLANCE

Problem Statement:

Despite growing awareness about oral health, a large segment of the population continues to delay dental care. Based on a mixed-method study involving 300 participants from Muradnagar, India, this book investigates the psychological, social, and systemic barriers that prevent timely dental visits. This behavior leads to worsened oral health outcomes, increased emotional distress, and greater long-term treatment costs, affecting not only individuals but also burdening the healthcare system as a whole.

Research Basis:

Using validated psychometric tools (MDAS, PSS, IPS) and the Kuppuswamy Socio-Economic Status Scale, the study collected data on anxiety, stress, procrastination, and socio-economic factors. A significant portion of respondents (93.4%) admitted to delaying dental care, influenced mainly by psychological stress, perceived cost, fear, and a belief that care isn't necessary unless symptoms are severe. The methodology combined clinical insights, qualitative interactions, and a structured statistical analysis to uncover patterns in patient behavior.

Key Findings:

35.3% of participants showed high dental anxiety

55% experienced moderate stress

23% reported high stress

31% had high procrastination tendencies

Delay in treatment was linked most strongly to a lack of perceived necessity

Females were more affected by procrastination and anxiety than males

Systemic Impact:

Delays in care have a cascading effect on public health. They increase the risk of chronic oral conditions, escalate treatment costs, and put additional strain on the healthcare system. Emotional barriers like shame, fear, and denial often go unnoticed, further deepening the silence around dental health. This silence isn't just emotional—it's economic, cultural, and systemic.

Recommendations:

1. For Healthcare Providers: Implement empathy-driven protocols, emotional architecture in clinics, and patient readiness tools.
2. For Policymakers: Adopt the 3A policy lens and invest in community-based dental workers (like the "Dental Didi" model).
3. For Technologists: Design multilingual, low-bandwidth tools that prioritize emotional safety and accessibility.
4. For Public Health Planners: Focus on behavior-based outreach, design-based dignity, and trust-centric healthcare delivery.

TABLE OF CONTENTS

Understanding Silence

Oral health is often one of the most neglected aspects of overall well-being. Not because people don't value it—but because it's surrounded by silence, hesitation, and a fair bit of misunderstanding.

This book doesn't aim to educate in the conventional sense. Instead, it tries to bring to light the hidden layers behind delayed dental visits, ignored pain, and hesitant conversations. Through real encounters, stories from camps and clinics, and reflections from the field, it explores how cultural beliefs, fears, accessibility, and awareness (or lack thereof) shape our choices around oral care.

Each chapter follows a narrative format—some reflective, some conversational—but all rooted in experiences that are common yet often overlooked. The goal isn't to preach solutions, but to start conversations.

In the coming pages, you'll journey through stories of patients who waited too long, caregivers who didn't know better, and settings—from rural campgrounds to polished OPDs—that show us the very real gap between clinical dentistry and patient reality.

Let's explore the unspoken together.

1.

The Dental Dilemma: Why We Delay Care

"We suffer more often in imagination than in reality."
— Seneca

There's a quiet space in every clinic—a moment that happens just before a patient opens up. It's not always visible, but it's there: in the eyes that avoid contact, in the gentle smile that masks uncertainty, in the sentence that trails off with a "maybe later."

I've stood in that moment many times.

At a dental camp in Muradnagar, I met a woman in her forties—draped in a fading pink dupatta, nervous fingers twirling the edge of her kurti. She hadn't come for treatment, she said. *"She asked me to tag along. That's all.."* But I offered her a seat anyway, and slowly, with hesitation softened by trust, she admitted, *"There's a tooth... It's been bothering me for some time. I thought it would go away."*
This wasn't unusual. It was familiar. Too familiar.

A boy of sixteen once told me he hadn't seen a dentist since childhood because he was scared his friends would laugh at his crooked teeth. A young mother, only twenty-eight, whispered, *"I haven't had time. Kids, work, home... I just keep postponing it."* An elderly man, sixty-seven, came in only when the pain became unbearable. *"Beta, I thought it was just old age. Why trouble you for this?"*

Different lives. Same thread.
A pattern woven through stories, sighs, and silences.

We often think dentistry is about the mouth.
But really, it's about the person behind it.
What they carry. What they hide. What they postpone.

Sometimes, people don't visit the dentist because they don't think they deserve the time or expense. Sometimes, they're too busy surviving the day. And often, they're just scared.

We judge people for not taking care of themselves, but rarely ask why they struggle to begin.

Procrastination is not laziness. It's often fear in disguise. Fear of pain. Fear of judgement. Fear of cost.

Or simply, the fear of finding out something might be wrong.

A woman in my study once said, *"I didn't delay because I didn't care. I delayed because I cared too much and didn't want to hear how bad it had gotten."*
That line stayed with me.
Because procrastination isn't carelessness—it's emotional self-protection.

The Role of Upbringing and Normalization

In many Indian homes, we're taught to endure. *"Thoda bardasht kar lo."* We apply this to pain, to fatigue, to ourselves. But we forget—endurance is not the same as self-respect.

Even in educated families, I've heard things like, *"My parents never took me to the dentist. We just got used to managing."*
Prevention isn't always seen as necessary. Pain is tolerated. And somewhere between resilience and resignation, our health is quietly compromised.

One of the most common beliefs I've encountered is about milk teeth. In several rural and even urban homes, parents don't bring their children to a dentist because *"yeh daant toh gir jaayenge."* They assume treatment isn't required for temporary teeth. What gets ignored is the potential for infections, the impact on permanent teeth, and the habits that are formed—or never formed—because early care was skipped.

Rural and Urban Camps – A Tale of Two Silences

In rural OPDs, I've noticed a recurring pattern. Patients don't come to the camp initially. Even those who do arrive, often want complete treatment right there—then and there. Referring them to a hospital becomes a challenge because travel isn't always feasible. The reasons are understandable: time, distance, money, trust.

In urban camps, the response is more open. Patients show up willingly—curious, even hopeful. But many are simply there for a diagnosis. *"Mujhe bas dekhna hai kya problem hai,"* they say. They just want to know. They don't always plan to act on it.

I remember one camp in a well-maintained society hall. Clean, organized, with polite families asking detailed questions—yet even here, many left without any intention of follow-up. Maybe it was fear, or cost, or convenience. But the silence was the same—just wrapped differently.

Notes from the Field

(Chamunda Chowk, Summer Afternoon)

A camp set under a tall peepal tree, the kind with rustling leaves that sound like whispers. Behind us flowed a narrow stream, its surface glinting in the sun. In front, the dusty road of the village stretched lazily. I remember how some patients didn't even approach the tent at first. They stood afar, watching.

But slowly, drawn in by the sight of others being heard, not hurried—they stepped closer. A man handed us chai in kulhads. Someone brought homemade ladoos, soft and warm. We didn't ask. They just gave.

Not everyone came for treatment. But many came to feel seen. That too, is healing.

Unseen Barriers

People delay dental visits for reasons that go beyond the obvious:

"I didn't want my husband to know I was spending on myself."
"I thought they'd judge me for how bad my teeth are."
"I've been meaning to go. I just don't know where the time goes."

These aren't excuses. These are emotions.
And every one of them is valid.

Some fear the financial implications. Others dread being scolded for neglect. Many are simply overwhelmed. Dental care is not always seen as urgent—until it is.

Empathy Before Everything

This book was not born in a lab.
It was born from these conversations.
From the warmth of trust. From the quiet tears in a dental chair.

From the guilt some patients carry and the love they show by showing up—even late.

I may be early in my journey, but I carry the voices of everyone I've met.
And I write this not to inform, but to connect.
Not to lecture, but to reflect.

Because behind every delay is a reason.
And behind every reason is a person trying their best.

If you've ever delayed care because life got busy, or fear held you back—you are not alone.
And if you're someone who cares for others—this is a window into what they may never tell you, but always feel.

Procrastination is a soft fog.
It whispers: "You still have time."
But health, like a sunrise, doesn't wait.
It asks us to rise before the day slips away.

2.

I'll Go Tomorrow: The Psychology of Procrastination

"Never put off till tomorrow what you can do the day after tomorrow just as well."
— Mark Twain

The Camp's Arrival in Sikri Kalan

Sikri Kalan, a small village tucked away in the heart of rural India, was the kind of place where life moved at its own pace, unaffected by the hustle and bustle of urban life. The air was thick with the smell of earth and dew, and the golden glow of the setting sun made everything seem timeless.

Simple homes, constructed from mud and thatch, dotted the landscape, blending effortlessly with the surrounding fields of crops. The village felt like a place untouched by the modern world, and yet, here we were, bringing a slice of that world to them.

The camp was set up in the village's central gathering spot, where the villagers would come together for celebrations, and now, it would host something a little different—a mobile dental van.
The van, a practical yet unassuming vehicle, brought with it the promise of care that the villagers hadn't experienced before. As the van arrived, it was met with a mixture of curiosity and hesitation.
The sight of dental chairs, machines, and tools was foreign to the residents of Sikri Kalan, many of whom had never seen such equipment up close.

But the camp was not just a chance to treat toothaches—it was a chance to show the villagers that dental care wasn't a luxury but a necessity for good health. It was a chance to break through the hesitation, to start a conversation about oral health that was long overdue.

"Tomorrow Never Comes"

As we started setting up the camp, a group of women stood nearby, quietly observing the preparations. Among them was Rukmini, a woman in her forties who had been suffering from a severe toothache for months. Despite her visible discomfort, she hadn't sought treatment. Meena, another woman, nudged her and said, *"Why don't you go? They can help with that pain."*

Rukmini hesitated, casting a long glance at the van. *"Maybe later,"* she said, though this wasn't the first time she'd said those words. *"I think it's just a small issue. Nothing serious."*

Meena was quick to respond,
"But it's been hurting you for weeks! You've said 'tomorrow' every day. What's really stopping you?"

Rukmini sighed, her eyes shifting away.
"I'm worried about the cost, Meena. And the time—it takes too long to go all the way to the camp. Who will take care of my field?"

It was a common hesitation. The reasons were practical—time, cost, and wary of unfamiliar spaces. But underlying these excuses was a deeper issue: a lack of trust. The village's healthcare system had always been based on traditional remedies, passed down through generations.

The idea of seeing a "city doctor" with modern equipment was both unfamiliar and intimidating.

Meanwhile, a conversation from the urban side echoed in my mind. Just a few weeks ago, I had a similar discussion with a friend in the city.

"I'll Deal With It Later"

"Don't you feel weird about going to the dentist? I always put it off. I know I should go, but there's always something else to do."

"Yeah, I get that. I had an appointment booked last week, and I canceled at the last minute. Too much work, you know?"

"Well, at least we have dentists just around the corner. You should go! It's not like we're in some village with one dentist every 100 miles."

It struck me how the same hesitation existed in both worlds, even if for different reasons. In the urban context, it was often about convenience or time. In rural areas, it was about trust, fear, and misinformation.

Delaying Care: A Universal Problem

The conversation between Rukmini and Meena wasn't unique. It was a reflection of a much broader issue that I had encountered in my time working in rural areas—people consistently putting off necessary care. The delay was not always due to a lack of access, but often because people felt that tomorrow would be soon enough.

It was a cultural mindset, a postponement that ran deeper than just dental care. Whether it was toothaches, fevers, or minor injuries, rural communities often preferred to wait and see if the problem would go away on its own. In urban settings, we are more accustomed to seeking quick medical attention for even the smallest of health issues.

But in places like Sikri Kalan, there was a prevailing belief that most health problems would resolve themselves with time, or that they weren't severe enough to justify immediate attention.

This tendency to wait until the problem became unbearable was something I had seen time and again. When it came to health, many people in rural areas treated it as a slow-moving, secondary priority, putting it on the backburner until it couldn't be ignored anymore.

Fears, Myths, and Misinformation

As the day wore on, more villagers gathered, each with their own stories of delayed dental care. Some had mild discomfort, others had severe issues, but all shared the same hesitation.

The wary of unfamiliar spaces was palpable. The mobile dental van, with its shiny, modern tools, seemed like something out of a sci-fi movie to many.

The villagers were accustomed to herbs, oils, and homemade remedies, but a dentist? That was something else.

One elderly man, who had been listening intently to the discussions, spoke up, *"I heard the dentists pull teeth without asking. What if they hurt me?"*

His comment was echoed by a few others, their expressions a mix of skepticism and fear. It wasn't just the unfamiliarity of modern dentistry that held them back—it was the misinformation they had heard from others.

"I heard it's very expensive," one woman added. *"And what if something goes wrong?"*

These fears weren't unfounded—they were based on stories, rumors, and the general mistrust that often accompanies new practices. In rural areas, where word-of-mouth carried a lot of weight, misinformation could spread quickly. There was a deep-seated concern that any treatment would come with side effects or, worse, that they would be left worse off than before.
In contrast, the urban side had its own set of worries, albeit more centered around convenience and finances.

Urban Realities: "Maybe Tomorrow?"

"I just don't have the time for all that dental checkup stuff. There's always a meeting or a project deadline. I'll go next week, I promise."

"Yeah, I keep telling myself the same thing. It's just... well, you know how it is in the city, right? Always on the go. And don't even get me started on the bills—dentists charge so much these days!"

"You can't let the cost scare you. It's your health, after all."

The hesitation was nearly identical. Whether in the village or the city, the underlying fears—of time, cost, and inconvenience—created barriers to seeking care.

The Reluctance to Let Go: A Deeper Reflection

I couldn't help but reflect on how similar this reluctance was to something more universal: the hesitation we all feel when faced with making an important decision. Whether it's health, finances, or relationships, we often put things off, telling ourselves that "tomorrow" will be better.

It's the same feeling when we know we should make an appointment but somehow convince ourselves that we can handle it later.

But here's the thing:
"Tomorrow" never comes until it absolutely has to. It's only when the pain is too much to ignore, when the situation becomes unbearable, that we finally take action.

This was true not only for the people in Sikri Kalan but for many of us in the modern world. We delay, we hesitate, we wait—until we can't.

The Power of Today

Despite all the hesitation and the delays, something powerful happened that day at the camp. Slowly, as the hours passed, people began to change their minds.
The once-skeptical villagers walked into the mobile van with tentative steps, unsure of what to expect but willing to try.
One by one, people sat in the dental chairs, and the fear began to dissolve.

The process wasn't just about fixing teeth; it was about breaking the cycle of hesitation, about showing people that care didn't have to be a painful, scary experience. The women who had initially hesitated were now helping others, guiding them toward the dental van, reassuring them that it wasn't as bad as they had feared.

Even Rukmini, who had promised herself she would go "tomorrow," finally made her way to the van. Her fear didn't vanish completely, but with each step she took, the idea of waiting faded away. And when her treatment was finished, the relief on her face was unmistakable.

Tomorrow is Today

As the camp wound down and the sun began to set over Sikri Kalan, I found myself reflecting on the day. The villagers' hesitation wasn't unique to them—it was something I had witnessed in cities, too, albeit for different reasons.

People were afraid of change, of the unknown, and of things they didn't fully understand. But the real breakthrough came not when we offered treatment—it came when we helped them overcome their fear and took that first step toward change.

We can always say "I'll go tomorrow," but the truth is that tomorrow never comes unless we make it happen today. And sometimes, all it takes is a little nudge, a little reassurance, and a little trust in something new to make that "tomorrow" become a reality.

If you've delayed care, I want you to know something.

You're not late.
You're not failing.
You're just human.

And being human means some days are heavy.
Some decisions are slow.
But even the smallest action, taken with love, can begin to melt the weight of waiting.

So tonight, maybe don't book the appointment.
Just whisper to yourself: *"I'm coming back to me."*
That alone is a beginning.

Delay is not indifference.
It's often unspoken tenderness toward ourselves—

A wish to feel safe before we feel healed.
But healing, too, can begin with a whisper.
A whisper that says, "Now is enough."

3.

What If It Hurts Again? – Memory, Fear, and Emotional Recall

"The body remembers what the mind forgets."
— A truth I've seen in every trembling hand that reaches for the dental chair.

There's a silence that speaks before any tool touches the mouth.
It lives in clenched fists, held breath, darting eyes.
In that moment, the dental chair becomes more than a seat—it becomes a place where fear returns home.

I've seen it in children.
In teenagers.
In adults with silver hair.

That subtle shift in posture. The way their fingers curl tightly into the armrest. The way their voice drops when they say, *"It's been a while."*

Fear has a language of its own—and over time, I've learned to hear it.

Dental fear is rarely about the sound of a drill.
It's about control. About memory. About not being ready the last time, and carrying that moment ever since.

The First Hurt Never Leaves Quietly

A woman in her early fifties once whispered, *"I was seven the first time. The dentist didn't tell me what he was doing. I felt pain, then pressure, then shame for crying. I've hated the smell of clinics ever since."*

She wasn't recalling a procedure—she was reliving a feeling.
Helpless. Unprepared. Small.

And it's not just her.

A college-going boy once sat stiffly in the chair and muttered, *"I'll be fine, I've had worse."* But the moment I picked up the mirror, his leg started shaking uncontrollably. I asked him gently, *"Would you like me to explain each step as we go?"* He paused. Then quietly said, *"No one has ever asked me that before."*

It's funny, isn't it? How we outgrow shoes, clothes, entire cities—but never outgrow emotional memories.

When the Mind Heals but the Body Doesn't Forget

In psychology, they call it Emotional Memory.
In real life, we call it a sinking feeling in your stomach.

The body is a quiet archive. It holds every gasp, every flinch, every time we were told to "be brave" when we weren't ready.
So even years later, under white light and clean gloves, the body whispers: "I remember."

And we freeze—not because we're weak, but because we were once hurt when we couldn't protect ourselves.
I once had a middle-aged man who looked like he could lift a car. Tough exterior, booming voice, business-like tone. But the moment I reclined the chair, he sat up again.

"I'm sorry," he said, embarrassed. *"I don't know why I'm reacting like this."*

"You're not reacting," I said. *"You're remembering."*

The Real Procedure is Emotional

Fear is the patient that enters before the real patient does.

A little boy once sat in my chair, tears forming before I even touched an instrument. His father stood beside him, saying, *"Don't be silly, it won't hurt."*
But I knelt beside him and said instead, *"It's okay to be scared."*

And in that moment, I saw his shoulders lower—not because the fear vanished, but because he was no longer alone in it.

There's no anesthesia for emotional pain.
But there is understanding.
Reassurance.
A warm light in a cold room.

Small Conversations, Big Walls

Once, during a community camp, I met a woman from a rural village who needed a simple extraction. Her pain was visible.
"You'll feel better after this," I told her.
She hesitated. Then whispered, *"Last time... my neighbor bled for two days. I am already anaemic, I don't want to die."*

Fear is shaped not just by memory, but by community memory—what others have said, suffered, or exaggerated.

A young software engineer in Delhi once said to me, *"I've read reviews... I know some dentists just overdo it for the money. I'm not ready to be scammed."*

Same fear, different masks.
One shaped by rumor, another by cynicism.
Both rooted in mistrust, both demanding more than just a treatment plan—they require rebuilding faith.

What If It Hurts Again?

That's the real question behind every delay.

Not *"will it hurt?"*
But *"what if I feel that same helplessness again?"*
"What if I cry again?"
"What if this time, I can't handle it?"

One patient said to me, *"I've been carrying this wisdom tooth pain for months. But the thought of sitting in that chair again... it gives me anxiety for days. I had a near death experience last time and I couldn't close my mouth"*
– apparently she had undergone a surgical wisdom tooth extraction and suffered from trismus (lock jaw) which is very common if mouth is kept wide open for very long.

We often mistake procrastination for laziness.
It's not.
Sometimes, it's armor.

"I'll go later" becomes a coping strategy.
A whisper of hope that today won't have to be the day we relive what we once barely survived.

A Different Kind of Strength

Sometimes, bravery isn't loud. It doesn't come wearing capes.
It arrives as someone walking through the clinic door after years of absence.
It speaks in voices that tremble and still say, *"Okay, let's try."*

One woman told me, *"I kept telling myself I'd come after my daughter's wedding. Then after my husband retired. Then after I got promoted. But really... I was waiting for the fear to disappear. It never did."*

I smiled and replied, *"That's okay. You didn't wait for the fear to go—you came anyway. That's braver.*

The Body Keeps the Score...
But It Also Writes New Ones

Healing doesn't begin with a scalpel.
It begins with trust.
And sometimes, a little bit of philosophy.

Maybe we're all just grown-up versions of children who once got hurt and never quite figured out how to say it out loud.

Maybe the mouth isn't just for chewing or speaking—but for holding back words we were never ready to say:
"I'm scared."
"I don't trust you yet."
"Please go slow."

The truth is, every appointment is two procedures—one physical, and one invisible.

And sometimes, the latter takes longer.

So what if it hurts again?

Then we breathe.
We pause.
We hold a hand, adjust the light, slow our pace.

We don't promise it won't hurt.
But we do promise that this time… they won't go through it alone.

*"Fear is the memory the body keeps.
Healing is the memory we create next."*

4.

She Just Came With Her Sister – The Moment of Readiness

"Change often begins quietly. In a breath, a sigh, a softened shoulder. Not in the doing—but in the willingness to finally begin." —Maggie Smith

She came to the camp wearing uncertainty like a shawl—folded tight, eyes lowered. Her sister filled out the form. She stood nearby, watching. Listening.

Her dupatta was wrapped twice around her shoulders like a protective shell. Her slippers were slightly worn, her hair oiled and neatly tied. The sister, on the other hand, had her kurta sleeves rolled up confidently and joked with the volunteer while filling in both their names.

"She insisted I come along.," the girl said softly, barely above a whisper.
I smiled and nodded.

As I moved on to attend to others, I kept sensing her presence near the edge. There's a kind of silence that isn't empty—it's brimming. That's how it felt.

Ten minutes later, her voice returned, smaller this time:

"Can you just take a quick look?"

That's where change begins. Not with declarations. But with tiny moments of courage wrapped in hesitation.

I've seen this shift hundreds of times—under tarps in community camps and in the air-conditioned quiet of a dental hospital. It doesn't matter where it happens. The decision to step forward is always sacred.

Behavioral science calls it "The Readiness Stage"—a mental tipping point. But to me, it's more poetic than that. It's not a stage.
It's a feeling.
A warmth.
A crack of light inside the heart.
And it rarely arrives from pressure. It grows in safe places.

She sat. I could sense her stillness as something earned.
Her hands gripped the side of the chair a little too tightly.
Her knees stayed pressed together.
I started gently.
"Just checking. Nothing scary."

She gave a tiny nod.

As I leaned in, I noticed her glance at her sister—who was already laughing with my colleague.

Even within families, readiness blooms differently.

Her molar needed treatment—but her spirit needed tending too. So I softened every word. And every movement. Because sometimes, it's not the extraction or cleaning that matters—it's how safe someone feels in that chair.

She hadn't just come for a check-up.
Maybe she came to finally be heard.
Maybe she came to see if she could still trust someone.
Maybe she came to prove something to herself.

Readiness doesn't always look like bravery. Sometimes it looks like showing up, softly.

She glanced at the chair like it held both fear and hope.

I imagined her thoughts—those questions we all carry:
"Will it hurt?" "What will they think?" "Will I be able to open my mouth properly?"
Or maybe something deeper: *"Can I trust this space?"*

And somewhere in that moment, she chose yes.

Three months earlier, at a camp held in a residential society in Raj Nagar, Ghaziabad, I met a man in his early 40s. Business suit, polished shoes, aviators resting on his forehead. From a distance, he looked like someone who had it all together.

He walked up briskly, hands in pockets. *"Just looking around,"* he said casually. I nodded.

I noticed him linger near the registration desk. He asked a student, *"Yeh sab kaun kar raha hai?"* (Who's doing all this?) The student explained about the outreach. He nodded again, then walked away.

Twenty minutes later, he came back.

"Actually... just a quick consult," he said, avoiding eye contact.

We sat down. He told me he hadn't seen a dentist in over a decade.

"Not scared. Just... kept postponing. Didn't seem urgent." Then, after a pause: *"But today... felt like I should show up. Don't know why."*

We started the check-up. His gums were inflamed, but treatable.

As we finished, he exhaled deeply and said, *"Thanks. I didn't even realise how tense I was."*

He stood up taller when he left. A small shift. A silent victory.

That moment reminded me: readiness doesn't belong to any gender, age, or income group. It arrives when the world finally feels quiet enough inside to take the next step.

It made me reflect how people can carry years of postponement—not because they don't care—but because they don't feel ready. And when readiness finally arrives, it comes in quietly, asking for a seat. An intern once told me, *"There was a boy who stood behind a tree the whole time. The next day, he came back—with his grandmother."*

Near the registration desk, I overheard two women whispering: *"Tu jaayegi?" "Nahi yaar, bas poochhne aayi hoon."*

Or a mother reassuring her son in the waiting line: *"Doctor gussa nahi karenge. Tum bas muh kholo, main yahin hoon."*

These murmurs matter. They form the emotional background music of every camp—the sound of fear turning slowly into trust.

With time, I've learned to notice the tiny cues—the way someone folds their arms tighter when you ask a question, or how their eyes soften when you smile. That's when I know they're ready, even if they haven't said a word.

Another intern said, *"I can tell who's ready. They walk around a few times before asking anything. And they always look at the chair like it's a mountain."*

He smiled. *"But when they sit... they always sit a little straighter after."*

That's the thing. Change happens in posture too. In how we hold ourselves once we feel seen.

Sometimes, people don't step forward for care because they feel they're not important enough. That their pain is too minor, their concern too silly. But every concern is valid. Every small discomfort matters.

I've come to believe that the first act of readiness is deciding: I matter enough to be helped.
One day, during a break, a woman approached holding a plastic bag with all her prescriptions.

"I know this is a dental camp," she said, *"but can I just talk to someone?"*

She wasn't asking for a tooth check. She just wanted to be heard. And that too, is readiness—to ask, to share, to not carry the weight alone.

That's why these camps matter—not just for diagnosis, but for what they awaken.
Sometimes readiness looks like finally applying for that job. Or walking away from someone who doesn't treat you right. Or deciding you'll try again—even if you failed the last time.

And often, the world doesn't celebrate these shifts because they look small on the outside.

But inside? They're monumental.
Back in the camp, the younger sister finally smiled as I reassured her.

"It's okay. We'll go slow."

She nodded again. A full nod this time.
The elder one grinned.

"Dekha? Told you it's nothing."

The younger girl didn't say anything. But she smiled back.
It was small.
And it was everything.

So, if you're reading this and waiting for the right moment in your lives—it may already be here.
The moment doesn't need to be grand.
It just needs to be yours.

"Readiness isn't about being fearless. It's about believing you're finally worth the care."

5.

When the Numbers Speak – What My Research Revealed

"The most important thing in communication is hearing what isn't said."
— Peter Drucker

When I looked at the data, I didn't just see percentages.
I saw pain.
I saw people who once said, *"I'm fine,"* when they weren't.
Over 93% of the individuals in my research study had delayed dental care. For many, the delay wasn't due to absence of pain, but due to presence of fear, shame, misinformation, and inaccessibility.

But numbers alone can't hold the weight of what I witnessed.
Each ticked box had a story.
Each answer was a sigh released after years of silence.

During my internship, I was a day scholar. Each morning, as I settled into the car, I'd rest my head on the windowpane and watch the world pass by. Normally, I'd fall asleep in minutes. But during the months of my research, I stayed wide awake. My mind spun with questions: Where are we going today? What kind of patients will I meet? How can I be softer, more patient, more present than yesterday?

Evenings were no different. On the drive back, the voices of the day stayed with me. Some hopeful. Some hesitant. Some still ringing with questions. Their faces lingered in my mind like familiar pages in a worn-out book.

The research started with a simple idea.
Idea to understand why people delay dental care. But when I began crafting the questionnaire, I realized how layered this question really was. I revised it many times. The aim was not to offend, but to gently peel back the hesitation.

Pilot testing helped. I asked friends, teachers, and a few patients to go through it. The feedback guided me: make it softer here, clearer there. But the real challenge came in the field—when I met people who couldn't read.
In such cases, I became the questionnaire.

I explained the purpose of the survey, assured them it was anonymous, and then asked each question slowly.
Not just for comprehension, but to build trust.
You can't rush trust.

And once it arrived, the truth poured in like rain.

One of the earliest camps we held was in Kachchi Sarai, a modest village where silence speaks louder than words. A woman in her 80's walked in—her gait weak, supported by two companions. She handed me a yellow camp card, the kind that allows economically vulnerable patients to avail treatment. I wondered why she had come to a dental camp when she looked like she needed a hospital bed.

We helped her into the chair. I asked her to open her mouth. And I froze.

Her teeth were all intact, yes. No decay, no caries.
But the bone had given up.
Her jaw had completely resorbed.
Her teeth, unsupported, danced like keys on an old piano.

They could be plucked out like flowers. And yet, she smiled with pride.

"Main roz tambaaku chabati hoon," she said.
She believed tobacco had preserved her teeth.

What it had actually done was rob her of nourishment. She hadn't eaten solid food in months. Her body had withered. But her faith in a myth remained unshaken.

I think of her sometimes. Her pride. Her frailty. The way she held onto belief when her body had nothing else left to hold. Her story stays with me, reminding me that numbers may fill a page, but it's empathy that fills the gap.

In Sanjay Colony, an urban locality, a young man came just to look around. He stood near the registration desk, reading the posters. *"I don't need anything. Just came with a friend,"* he said. But he lingered.

After twenty minutes, he returned.

"Maybe you can just check," he said, avoiding eye contact.

His gums were inflamed.
Teeth were missing.
Visible deep cavities.
Because of missing teeth, remaining changed their position.
And what not.
He hadn't seen a dentist in over ten years. Not because he didn't care—but because it never felt urgent enough.

"It's not like I was in pain," he explained. *"But I guess... I kept waiting."*

He's not alone. Many wait. For pain. For time. For courage.

But the cost of delay isn't just medical. It's emotional. And sometimes, social.

A young woman I met had withdrawn completely from social life. Her complaint? Chronic bad breath.

"I brush twice. I rinse. I do everything right. Still, people step back when I speak."

She had stopped meeting friends. Avoided gatherings. Her smile was always closed-lipped. Her self-worth had become tied to a condition she couldn't explain.

In another camp, a boy no older than eight sat with his shoulders curled. I asked him gently, *"Dard ho raha hai?"*
He nodded. But when I asked if he had told his mother, he looked away.

"Mummy daantengi," he whispered.

He feared punishment more than pain.

Back at the hospital one day, I met a frail elderly man who had once tried to pull out his tooth using a metal wire. It hurt for weeks, and he had no access to care. But he didn't come to a dentist. He thought pain was a part of old age. Something to be endured.

These aren't just stories. These are truths buried behind delay.

When I sat down to analyze the results of my study—over 300 people surveyed, across rural and urban settings—the numbers aligned with the faces.
93.4% had delayed dental care.

Over 60% showed signs of moderate to severe dental anxiety.

Psychological stress, procrastination, and poor oral health habits were closely linked.

But a stat like "60%" doesn't show you trembling hands or darting eyes. It doesn't reveal the boy who hides his pain. Or the pride of a woman built on brittle teeth.

It doesn't show the silence.

Numbers can only whisper. Stories let them sing.

Sometimes, I think back to the apartment camp at River Heights in Rajnagar Extension. A posh setting. Neat lawns. Educated residents. Yet, even there, I heard the same phrases:

"I kept delaying." "Didn't think it was important." "I was scared of the tools."

The address changes. The fears remain.

Many patients weren't just avoiding dentists—they were falling through the cracks of a system that never reached them.

One afternoon, as we returned from a long camp day, I sat in the car, watching sunlight flicker through dusty glass. I wasn't tired—I was full. Full of faces. Of smiles. Of fears. Of strength. I rested my head and wondered: How many more are out there, hurting quietly?

The ripple of this study didn't stop when I tallied the final numbers.
It didn't end with the last submission form or the printed certificate.
It stayed with me—in the subtle shift of my posture when a hesitant patient walks in.
In the way I slow down my explanations now, not just to inform, but to comfort.

This research taught me that numbers are not a destination.
They're a beginning.
A map that only makes sense when you travel it with empathy.

I began noticing things more deeply: the pause before a patient answers, the glance toward the door, the way someone grips the chair just a little too tightly.

These details—often invisible in a graph—became louder than data.

When I sit across from someone now, I no longer see "a case."
I see a story unfolding—quiet, cautious, full of history.

And I ask myself:
How can I make this a moment where they feel safe enough to continue that story?
That's the real power of reflection.
Not to record what was, but to reshape what will be.
Because if a study ends in a journal, it's simply read.
But if it ends in your behavior, your intention, your voice—it lives.

This research didn't just make me a better clinician.
It made me a deeper listener.
A softer presence.
A witness to the unspoken.
This chapter is not just about data.
It is about people.
About pain hidden behind politeness.
About voices that finally chose to speak.

Irving Selikoff rightly said that:

> *"Statistics are people with the tears wiped off."*

6.

Not Just a Toothache – The Hidden Weight of Stress

"The mouth is a mirror of the body, and sometimes, of the mind."
– Unknown

She walked in slowly, pressing her palm gently against her cheek, as if to muffle the pain or hide it from the world.

Her name, age, gender, complaint—all filled in on the card.
Under 'Chief Complaint': *Toothache.*

But what followed told me it wasn't just that.

I looked up and saw a young woman, maybe in her early thirties, sitting on the edge of the chair like she was ready to run. Her eyes were tired—not the tiredness that comes after a long day, but the kind that settles in after a long year.

"Since when?" I asked, gently.

She thought for a moment.

"More than a year," she said. *"But I thought it would go on its own."*

She wasn't lying. She genuinely believed that pain had an expiry date.

I've learned that when people say *"It's just a toothache,"* they rarely mean the pain is small.

What they really mean is: *I've learned to live with it.*

Toothaches aren't always emergencies in their world. They are interruptions. Background noise. Something to ignore until it demands attention.

And when it does, it isn't just about the tooth anymore. It becomes about missed meals, broken sleep, snapped tempers, and silent suffering.

I once met an elderly man who came to a rural camp in Ballabgarh. He had swelling near his jaw and a deep, persistent ache. His son brought him in after weeks of persuasion.

"He's not eating," the son told me. *"Says nothing is soft enough."*

I asked the man how long it had been hurting.

"Six months," he said flatly.

I asked why he waited.

He shrugged. *"I thought it was gas. Or maybe a cold. These things happen with age."*

But it wasn't gas. It was a deep infection. And the body had been shouting long before the words caught up.

One camp in Rasulpur remains etched in my memory. A woman came wearing a red saree and a polite smile.

"Bas dard hai," she said.

When I examined her, I saw more than decay. Her gums were bleeding. Her tongue had ulcers. Her breath was heavy with infection.
I asked a few questions—about hygiene, habits, history. She hesitated.

Then said quietly, *"Main thak gayi hoon. Har waqt kuch na kuch chubhta hai muh mein. Par ab aadat si ho gayi hai."*

(I'm tired. There's always something hurting in my mouth. But I've gotten used to it now.)

That line settled in me. **"I've gotten used to it now."**

How many of us get used to discomfort, until it becomes our normal?

Pain is not always loud.
Sometimes, it's a whisper. A numbness. A heaviness that sits behind the eyes and makes everything feel slow.

There was a boy in Metro Homes, a quiet residential society. He was sixteen. Neat hair, slouched posture. He came in with his mother, who did all the talking.

"He says his teeth hurt. But I think he's just avoiding school," she said with a half-smile.
When I spoke to him alone, he said, *"It hurts when I chew. And I don't feel like eating anymore. I get headaches. I feel sleepy all the time."*

His case looked routine—a few cavities, some sensitivity. But his tone wasn't.

"Are you feeling okay otherwise?" I asked.

He looked away. *"Not really. But it's nothing. Just a toothache, right?"*

I paused.

Sometimes, the tooth is fine.
And the child is hurting.

I once had a patient in the hospital—a woman in her late forties. Her complaint was mild bleeding from the gums.

She was well-spoken, sharp, with a calm exterior. But her hands shook.

"Do you have any other health issues?" I asked.

She nodded slowly. Then whispered, *“Depression. I stopped brushing for months. Everything felt heavy.”*

The bleeding wasn’t the root problem.
It was the symptom of being tired. Of giving up.

She didn’t need just scaling. She needed someone to notice her.

This chapter isn’t about decay or disease.
It’s about the layers beneath them.

Toothache is rarely just about teeth.
It’s about all the things we keep delaying, denying, or swallowing.
It’s about grief. Shame. Fatigue.

It’s about survival.

In camps, people often come for check-ups but stay back to talk.

"Bas puchhne aaye the," they say.
But their eyes say something else.

They want to be seen. Heard. Reassured that pain is not weakness.
They want permission to feel what they've been numbing.

And sometimes, in that chair, the tooth becomes a doorway.

A doorway to conversations never had.
To care long denied.
To a sigh they didn't know they were holding.

I've come to believe that healing doesn't always begin with a prescription.
It begins with a pause.

With a question asked gently.
With a hand that doesn't rush.

Toothache, like many kinds of pain, is a messenger.
And behind every complaint is a story waiting to unfold.

"Pain always demands to be felt. But healing asks to be heard."

Through My Eyes

There are things I witnessed that no form could capture. Not the scales I filled, nor the data I recorded. Moments lived quietly—in the way a patient hesitated, or sat too slowly.

Those moments shaped me.

This isn't about statistics. It's about presence.
Being there when someone finally sits. Standing by while a woman speaks through silence. Listening to a story that was never fully told.

I remember the quiet between two sisters as one filled out a form. A boy who winced before I opened the tray. An elderly woman who walked miles just to ask, "Is it too late?"

In those moments, I wasn't a clinician. I was a witness.

You learn that people don't always need advice—they need someone who listens without flinching. Care doesn't begin with a diagnosis. It begins with a pause. With presence.

I've sat on village benches as strangers spoke without words. Their pain in metaphors, their emotions sitting beside them quietly.

In homes where illness is ignored, I saw quiet strength. Not dramatic, but the kind that rises each day, tends to life, and swallows pain.

I saw women who gave up meals before work. Men who cried only in solitude. Children who whispered fears no one else heard.

These are not textbook tales. They are windows. Windows into lives that trusted me with what was never said aloud.

This is what I saw. This is what stayed.
This is Through My Eyes.

7.

The Bench in the Camp, the Chair in the Clinic

"Where we sit shapes what we say. Sometimes the heart opens more easily under trees than under tubes."— Anonymous

There is something sacred about a wooden bench beneath a tree.

It doesn't have back support. It wobbles a little. Sometimes it creaks. But it carries stories.

In the camps, we often place these benches near our mobile vans. They are rarely empty.
Children sit there kicking their legs, elders rest their walking sticks against them, women gather in twos and threes—talking, watching, waiting.

These benches are not just for waiting. They are for softening.
They allow people to arrive in parts.

A woman may come and sit with no intent to be treated. Just to accompany someone. But while sitting, she watches. She listens. She gathers courage.

I remember one such camp in Muradnagar, a rural settlement flanked by fields and narrow lanes. We had set up our chairs under a mulberry tree, its fruit dotting the ground like little ink stains. The sun filtered through the leaves in golden streaks. The breeze carried sounds of cows, laughter, and distant temple bells.

A wooden bench stood a few feet from our van. That day, it felt like a confessional booth.

A girl in her twenties sat on it. Clutching her dupatta tightly. She hadn't registered.
She told a volunteer she had just come to see what was happening.

But as others around her went in, got examined, and returned, she stayed.
Then, after a long while, she walked up and said, *"Main baith sakti hoon?"* (Can I sit?)

She sat in the chair and looked straight ahead, not at me.

She had fluorosis — brown stains and pitted enamel.

"Shaadi nahi ho rahi," she said flatly. (I'm not getting married.)

Her voice cracked only once. *"Ek baar rishta pakka hua tha. Unhone mana kar diya."* (A match had been fixed. They rejected me.)

I examined her, gave her options for cosmetic management. But what she really needed that day was not just dental advice.
She needed to be witnessed.
She needed to say aloud the quiet grief she had been carrying.

And for that, the bench had done its work.

Not far from her, a little boy with dust on his cheeks sat cross-legged beside the bench, watching everything like it was a live drama.
"Doctor banoge?" I asked, teasing.

He giggled and shook his head. *"Mujhe bas yeh dekhna hai ki aap log dard dete ho ya nahi."*

He wasn't even a patient, but that moment reminded me: benches don't just hold patients. They hold observers. Watchers. Tomorrow's stories.

Two women on the bench were discussing their experiences:
"Tere daant dard karte hain?"
"Nahi yaar, par darr lagta hai. Machine chalti hai na andar."
They both laughed nervously.
That laughter was more than humor. It was collective courage.

The bench, in many ways, is like a waiting heart.
It doesn't push. It doesn't prescribe. It listens.
It holds people who don't know they're ready until they stand up and walk toward care.
It offers what medicine alone often can't: time.

The bench allows people to arrive as they are.
There is no expectation.
No mask.

People joke. They share home remedies. They ask others what happened inside the van. There is a sense of community healing, not just medical.
But in the clinic, the chair feels different.

The patient is alone.
The light is harsh.
The walls are white.

They are asked to open wide, to answer quickly, to comply.

Sometimes, I can see their shoulders rise as they sit.
Their fingers curl around the armrest.
Their lips press tight even before I speak.

Some cross their legs tightly. Others tap their fingers on the armrest. One man stared at the light the whole time, refusing to blink.

Our bodies speak before we do.
In clinics, they say: I don't know if I'm safe here.
On benches, they say: I'm watching. Deciding. Maybe I'll speak soon.

Once in our college clinic, a middle-aged man sat down with arms crossed.
He had been referred from a nearby satellite center.
His file said: *"Severe attrition. Multiple missing teeth. Needs partial denture."*

But he kept deflecting every question.
"Koi dikkat nahi hai. Bas formalities ke liye aaya hoon."
(There's no issue. I just came because they asked me to.)

It took several minutes before he admitted he hadn't eaten properly in months.
His gums hurt. His self-esteem was low.

He opened up slowly, cautiously, as if every sentence had to be tested for judgment.

In that white chair, under the buzzing light, vulnerability was harder.

In another camp in Sanjay Colony, a well-dressed woman came in with her teenage daughter.
"Just a regular cleaning," she said. But the daughter's body said otherwise—arms folded, chin tucked, eyes avoiding mine.

When I tried speaking directly to her, she gave short answers. Her mother answered for her.

The chair had made her feel small. Watched. Judged.

That day I realized—silence isn't always shyness.
Sometimes it's someone waiting for safety.

One man came in stiff, visibly tense. I noticed his phone wallpaper had a goat wearing sunglasses. I smiled and asked, *"Yeh aapka dost hai?"*

He laughed—loudly.
The grip on the armrest softened.
Sometimes the lightness of a question is stronger than anesthesia.

And yet, both spaces matter.

The bench is where hesitation breathes.
The chair is where action begins.

But we must carry the kindness of the bench into the chair.
We must let people arrive in layers, even in clinics.
We must speak like there's a tree above us, like the ground is still warm, like there are people around who understand.

Because no amount of sterilized trays can clean fear.
That needs presence.

I remember during internship, after a long day of OPD, I sat on one of the benches outside the hospital gates. A woman who had visited earlier in the day came and sat beside me.

"Maine pehle kabhi aise kisi se baat nahi ki," she said.

Not about her toothache, but about the loneliness she carried.
That evening, I realized—sometimes people don't return for treatment. They return for listening.

I often wish we could redesign clinics to feel more human.
To play the music of someone's language.
To smell like home.
To have windows.

I've sometimes imagined a future clinic—not with a reception counter behind glass and a queue of patients with tokens—but with a courtyard.
A space with light coming in through real windows, not frosted partitions.
Where waiting areas have comfortable seating.
Where walls aren't decorated with scary anatomical charts, but with drawings made by children who once sat in the chair and left a little braver than they came.

What if instead of saying *"next!"*, we said, *"Aayiye, baithiye"*?
What if, before picking up a probe, we offered a story?

The bench taught me that the best care doesn't start with examination. It starts with observation. With patience. With presence.
Maybe we can never fully replicate the shade of a mulberry tree in a dental cubicle. But we can carry its spirit.

That spirit—of comfort, slowness, conversation—is what we need most in the places where people open their mouths and often, their fears.

Because when someone lets you look inside their mouth, they're letting you into a deeply personal part of their life. It should feel like a moment of trust, not of tension. And that's why I say: the chair must borrow from the bench.

One is clinical. The other is emotional.
But healing requires both.

Until then, we carry the softness of the field bench inside our voices.
We become the tree that offers shade.

"Healing is not just about where it hurts, but where you feel safe enough to talk about it."

8.

Between Shame and a Smile

"Shame corrodes the very part of us that believes we are capable of change."
— Brené Brown

There is a moment I've come to recognize—a pause, subtle but profound—when someone is about to open their mouth for the first time in a dental camp or clinic. It's a flicker in the eyes, a glance toward the ground, a half-turn of the face. Not everyone shows fear. But many show shame.

Shame does not shout. It sits quietly, tucked between self-consciousness and silence.
It's in the way a woman adjusts her dupatta to hide her mouth when she laughs.
In how a child stares at the floor while speaking.
In the man who brings his nephew to camp but refuses to sit himself, saying, *"Mere daant toh theek hain,"* even when they clearly aren't.

It's not pain that holds people back. It's the belief that their pain makes them unworthy of help. It's not cavities or calculus that keep mouths closed—it's the thought that someone might judge them for having them.

The Camp in Sanjay Colony

It was an urban outreach camp, set up inside a gated housing colony. A plastic table, a folding chair, a banner flapping in the wind. The buildings had washed balconies and drying clothes waving like flags—domestic, colorful, human.

She arrived just before noon. Hair tied in a bun, a crisp dupatta, bangles that clinked as she folded her arms tightly across her chest. She was in her mid-thirties, and she looked like someone used to being composed. But when she sat, the composure cracked.

"I haven't smiled properly in years," she said, voice low. *"Even with my children. I keep my lips shut."*

She had gaps, discolored teeth, and deep periodontal pockets. She didn't want treatment that day. She just wanted to say it aloud.

That moment has never left me.
Sometimes, shame is not the fear of what others will say.
It's the sadness of what we've already told ourselves.
The quiet judgment we carry alone for too long.

She didn't want a mirror. She wanted understanding.
She didn't ask for help. She asked to be heard.
And in doing so—she began to smile again.

The Boy Whose Teeth Wore Clothes

He must've been in Class 8 or 9—skinny frame, oversized shirt, hair parted neatly to the side. He came to our satellite clinic with his mother, who sat beside him with folded hands and tired eyes.

When I asked what the issue was, she simply said, *"Aap ek baar dekh lijiye."*
The boy wouldn't look at me. He clutched the edge of the chair, knuckles pale.

I gestured gently, *"Come sit here."* He hesitated, then obeyed.

"Open your mouth, beta," I said softly.
He turned his face slightly. His lips trembled.
And then he opened.

What I saw took a second to register.

His teeth—top, bottom, front, back—were covered in a thick, dark, crusty mass of calculus. Not the kind you see in older patients. This looked like his teeth had worn stone armor, like they were dressed in layers of cement.

"Do you brush your teeth?" I asked gently.

He shook his head. *"Kabhi nahi."*

Not even once.

When I picked up the scaler, he flinched. *"Dard hoga,"* he muttered.
"Thoda hoga," I admitted. *"But not as much as the pain of carrying this forever."*

He squirmed, resisted. *"Aap daant tod doge,"* he whispered.

And honestly—it did feel like breaking stone.

Every stroke of the scaler scraped against hardened plaque that had lived there for years. It didn't flake off. It shattered.
"Toot gaya na daant!" he accused as tiny bits broke free.

"No, beta," I said with a smile. *"Tohfa de rahi hoon tumhare asli daant ka."*

He didn't laugh. But he stayed.

Only a quarter of the scaling was done that day. He was told to return for three more sittings.

He never came back.

Not the next day, not the next week. Not ever.

Sometimes, I wonder why.
Maybe it was the discomfort. Maybe the sensation of being exposed. Or maybe—just maybe—it was shame.

The kind that makes you feel you're too far gone to be fixed. The kind that whispers, *"Stay invisible. It's easier."*

I often imagine him walking home, lips pressed tightly, heart a little heavier. I imagine life swallowing him back into routine. The toothbrush still unused. The mouth still hiding.

And I wonder:

Did we fail to make the clinic feel safe enough?
Did his shame win?

The Girl in Yellow: Kachchi Sarai Rural Camp

I remember her clearly. A teenage girl wearing a mustard salwar-kameez, faded at the edges but clean and pressed. She had a notebook in her hand and clutched it to her chest like a shield.

She came with her aunt, who needed an extraction. The girl sat on the wooden bench and waited. Watching. Listening.

After her aunt was done, I asked gently, *"Tumhara check-up kara lein?"*

She shook her head. Then, after a pause, whispered,
"Daant ache nahi hain."
Her front incisors were brown. The enamel pitted.
Typical of fluorosis. When I asked if it hurt, she said no.

Then I asked why she never came before.

She looked at her feet. *"Log bolte hain muh se badbu aati hai. School mein sab chidhate hain."*

That sentence stayed with me. Not because it was uncommon—but because it was so heartbreakingly normal.

We gave her a free scaling. I explained her options. We didn't promise perfection. We promised care.

And when she got off the chair, her shoulders were straighter.
Just a little.
But enough.

Sometimes, healing doesn't start with medicine. It starts with a pause. A conversation. A space that says, You're welcome here. You're not disgusting. You're not broken. You're not alone.
Shame is a quiet prison.

Smile is the jailbreak.

Shame isolates. Smile connects.
Shame says, "Hide." Smile says, "Come forward."
Shame freezes you. Smile frees you.
I've come to believe that dental care, at its best, is not just clinical—it is deeply emotional work. The act of helping someone open their mouth is, more often than not, the act of helping them open a part of themselves they've hidden for years.

People don't always come to fix their teeth.
They come to see if they can still be seen.

And when they are met without judgment—when a clinic becomes a kind place, when a dentist becomes a listener—something shifts.

A woman walks out with her lips parted in relief.
A boy tastes the cold sting of air on a tooth long buried.
A girl finds out that her brown spots don't make her unworthy.

And none of them may laugh out loud. Not yet.

But they'll go home and maybe look at themselves a little differently.

They'll pick up the brush.
They'll start again.
Because they were seen.

Because someone told them—without words—*"You are still worthy of smiling."*

"Shame dies when stories are told in safe places...
And to be seen—not judged but gently held in that seeing—is the most terrifying, and the most beautiful thing."

9.

The Women I Sat With

"There is no force more powerful than a woman determined to rise."
— W.E.B. Du Bois

The camp that day was set under a neem tree in Meerapur. A makeshift bench had been laid out with plastic stools beside it. The morning sun hadn't fully risen, and dew still clung to the tall grass around the village pathway. In the distance, you could hear the clink of bangles, the clang of aluminum utensils, and the murmur of women speaking in soft voices, low and rhythmic like poetry passed between generations.

They arrived in groups—some with their children, others with their friends. Most walked slowly, sarees pulled over their heads, chappals worn thin. They didn't come for themselves.

They rarely do.

They came because someone told them a dental camp was happening. Because their neighbor insisted. Because their son or sister-in-law dragged them along. And they sat—quietly, patiently, holding their pain like folded laundry.

The Mother Who Didn't Speak

She must have been in her late forties.
Her saree was pale blue, her wrists full of glass bangles.
When asked why she had come, she smiled and said,
"Bas yunhi. Dekhne."

She sat with her hands tightly clasped in her lap. When I asked if anything hurt, she shook her head.

But something in her eyes didn't agree.

After a few minutes, as the camp quieted down, she leaned forward and whispered, *"Peechle do mahine se kuch bhi thanda nahi kha sakti."*

It wasn't just about the tooth. It was the fact that she had waited two months. That she had prioritized school fees,

hospital trips for her husband, and ration shopping over her own pain.
When I gently asked why she didn't come earlier, she looked down and said, *"Mere liye time kaun nikaalega?"*

The Widow Who Smiled Through the Pain

In a clinic in Ghaziabad, I once treated an elderly woman who had lost most of her teeth but still insisted she was doing fine.

"Daant ab kaun banwaata hai is umar mein?" she laughed. *"Bas do roti chaba leti hoon."*

Her gums were inflamed.
The sharp ridges of broken molars had left ulcers. But she smiled as if nothing hurt.
Only when I applied a little pressure did she wince.

"Thoda dard toh rehta hai, beta. Aadat si ho gayi hai."

Aadat.
Not a complaint. Just an adaptation.

The Girl in the Green Dupatta

She arrived last. She waited until the crowd had thinned out.
When she finally approached, she refused to sit. *"I just want to ask... kuch brown spots hain daanton pe... woh hat sakte hain kya?"*

As she spoke, her eyes darted. Her hands kept fidgeting with the hem of her dupatta.

She was twenty-one. She had fluorosis stains across her front teeth. She had been rejected by three prospective grooms.

"Nazar daanton pe hi jaati hai sabki," she said with a bitter laugh.

I told her the stains could be managed. She didn't smile, but she nodded.
Later, before leaving, she returned to say, *"Aap pehli doctor ho jinhone bina judge kiye baat ki."*

That sentence stayed with me for days.

The Young Daughter Who Translated

In Sultanpur, an elderly woman came in with her teenage daughter. The girl spoke, the mother didn't.

"She's had pain in the back tooth for months," the girl said.

When I asked the mother directly, she just smiled and looked at her daughter.

"Amma doesn't talk to doctors," the girl explained. *"Par aaj mein saath hoon."*

The daughter gave consent. The daughter asked questions. The daughter held her mother's hand during the extraction.

It was quiet strength. Inherited. Then returned.

A Group of Women

At a camp in the rural region of Guldhar, we had a plastic tarp laid over bricks and benches under a mango tree. It was humid, the air sticky with sweat and soap. A group of five women sat in a circle, sharing a single steel tiffin of parathas and chutney while waiting.

They laughed, joked, teased each other about their 'daant ki halat'—but when it came time for checkups, all of them suddenly grew quiet.

One got up, saying, *"Main pehle jaaungi. Agar theek laga toh tum log bhi aana."*

It wasn't the treatment they feared—it was being seen.

Each one came, eventually. They needed scaling, fillings, one needed an extraction. But what they needed most was each other. Their strength was shared. So was their silence.

And I realised—sometimes healing begins in a circle of women passing time, not in a chair.

The Woman Who Took Off Her Jewellery

In an urban satellite clinic, a woman in her thirties came in wearing bright bangles and a golden chain. Before sitting on the chair, she began removing everything slowly, methodically.

When I asked gently, *"Zarurat nahi hai, aap pehenke baith jaaiye,"* she laughed and said, *"Doctorji, yeh ladayi ke liye tayyari hai."*
We both laughed. And somehow, the treatment went smoother than expected.

Sometimes, humour becomes armour. And laughter, the first step towards trust.

The Reflection of My Own Silence

I remember a day during my internship. It was raining lightly outside, and we were returning from a camp. I sat by the window, forehead resting against the cool glass, watching the fields blur into green and brown streaks.

My thoughts were full—not of procedures, but of conversations.

The woman who whispered her pain. The girl who asked if her smile could be restored. The mother who said she'd come only for her daughter.

Every face sat beside me in that van. Every voice echoed in my chest.

I didn't just sit with these women during treatment. They sat with me afterward—in memory, in reflection, in all the small spaces between clinical facts and emotional truths.

Language, Silence, and Being Heard

Many of the women who came didn't have the words to explain their pain. They didn't know the names of their problems. Some didn't speak Hindi fluently. Some whispered in Bhojpuri or Awadhi, shy and unsure. And some simply pointed.

Pain isn't always loud. Sometimes, it arrives in gestures, in glances, in borrowed voices.

Learning to understand that has been as important as learning to treat.

A Quiet Revolution

They don't raise slogans. They don't shout their needs. But they show up—after cooking, cleaning, raising kids, caring for parents. They walk for kilometers. They sit quietly on benches. They apologize for bleeding gums and broken fillings, as if pain was their fault.

And yet, they stay.

They let strangers look into their mouths. They let strangers touch what they’ve been told to hide.

And that, to me, is bravery.

In My Diary

One entry says:

> “She said, ‘*Main toh bas uski saath aayi thi... par lagta hai mujhe bhi check kara lena chahiye.*’
I didn’t ask what changed her mind. I just handed her the bib.”

Another reads:

> “A mother came with four children and left only after each had seen a dentist.
When I asked if she wanted a check-up too, she said,
‘*Mere daant ka kya kaam hai? Main toh sirf sabko sambhalti hoon.*’”

That line made me pause.
Because she wasn't just referring to her teeth.
She was referring to her role.

The Silent Strength

I've come to realize—women don't delay treatment because they're careless. They delay it because they're too careful—with money, time, love, responsibility. Their own health falls last.

And when they finally sit in the chair, they bring all of that with them. Not just plaque and pain—but duty, fatigue, fear, guilt, hope.

We treat more than teeth. We treat silence. We treat sacrifice.

And we offer one quiet thing in return: Respect.

"How many women around us are waiting to be heard, not just healed?"

10.

Voices That Stayed With Me

"The human voice is the organ of the soul."
– Henry Wadsworth Longfellow

Some voices don't fade.

They echo in the quietest hours—between brushing and bedtime, in the spaces where memory sharpens.

Not because they were loud. But because they were true.

In every camp, in every clinic, I carried back more than patient details. I carried back voices.

"Mere daant ache hain, lekin main khush hoon."

She was 65, with a deep smile and a thin red bindi between her brows. Her saree had faded sunspots and her voice carried no complaint.

Her teeth, however, told another story. Severe attrition, mobile teeth, chronic infection.

"Pain toh hai, par aadat ho gayi."

There was something in the way she said it that didn't feel like resignation. It felt like she had found peace with her pain—like a woman who had held so much in life that now, a hurting molar was just one more thing to fold into her daily routine.

"Agar main chali gayi toh bacchon ka kya hoga?"

She had come from rural camp reference, after three refusals. Her children walked with her that day, barefoot. She sat quietly until everyone else had gone.

She had an abscess that needed urgent attention. But she was more worried about the recovery days.

"Main 4 din ke liye bhi bimar pad gayi toh sab bigad jaata hai."

It wasn't the pain that kept her from treatment. It was the burden of being the spine of her home.

Her voice was firm, yet laced with helplessness—a voice that had negotiated with life for too long.

"Kaash maine pehle aapko mil liya hota."

This one came from a woman who had lost most of her upper teeth due to a preventable infection.

She wasn't angry. She wasn't bitter.
She was grateful.
She said this while holding my hand after the consultation.

And her words weren't just about dentistry. They were about being seen. Heard. Held without judgment.
We don't always know what patients expect from us. But sometimes, they just want to feel safe.

"Doctor, muh kolne mein sharam aati hai."

A young woman in her twenties whispered this while cupping her hand around her mouth.

She worked in a garment factory. Fluorosis had turned her teeth patchy and yellow. A colleague once teased her. She hadn’t smiled since.

She had begun covering her mouth when she laughed, when she spoke, even when she yawned..
Her voice was muffled by shame. But her eyes were pleading.

We forget how much we use our mouth to live, to love, to express.
And when that becomes a source of embarrassment, it doesn’t just affect dental health.
It affects identity.

The Voice That Didn't Come from the Mouth

Sometimes, it's not what they say. It's what they don't.

The woman who brought her daughter but never said a word. The girl who came three times before sitting down. The old lady who nodded, but didn’t answer, until you asked her in Bhojpuri.

Silence can be a voice too. A heavy one. A loud one.

An Urban Clinic in Officer's City

I met a woman in a formal salwar suit, expensive handbag, perfectly threaded brows.

"Just a cleaning," she said.

As we spoke, it became clear she was dealing with years of bleeding gums and sensitivity.

"Mujhe dar lagta hai," she finally admitted. *"Kahin phir se woh pain na ho jaaye jo pehle hua tha."*
She had gone to a dentist years ago and had a traumatic extraction.

Her voice cracked.

"Main kisi ko nahi bata payi. Sab haste the."
Fear doesn't always wear tattered clothes. Sometimes it wears perfume and walks into urban clinics.

Whispers in the Camp

Some of the strongest voices come in hushed tones.

A girl barely twelve whispered, *"Mummy ne bola, daant dikhane se rishta nahi aayega."*

Another said, *"Main brush karti hoon roz, fir bhi muh se smell aata hai."*
Another sat beside her mother and spoke for both of them.

"Amma ke daant hil rahe hain, par woh dar rahi hain." She looked at me. *"Aap chillate toh nahi na?"*

That made me pause.

Because someone, somewhere, had made her believe that asking for care would invite anger.

After the Camps, the Echoes

When I return from camps, I hear their voices while lying on my bed.

Not out loud. But deep in the folds of memory.

Some voices are like prayers. Some like unfinished questions. Some, just silent exhalations of relief.

The Voice Within Me

I carry all these voices.

They return to me when I'm quiet. They guide me when I forget why I started. They keep me soft, especially on days when I'm tired, or hurried, or unsure.

I don't remember every name. But I remember the tone, the tremble, the truths they carried.

They remind me: We don't just treat mouths. We hold stories.

And every story told without fear is one step closer to healing.

A Voice That Changed Me

There was once a woman who, after a difficult extraction, said, *"Aap sab doctor log insaan bhi ho kya?"* and then laughed quietly.
I laughed too, but later, I cried.

Because her voice made me realize how deeply patients expect indifference. That simple question, asked half-jokingly, became my turning point.
Since then, I've tried every day not just to be a doctor, but to be human first.

A Voice I Heard Too Late

A teenage girl had come to a camp. She asked repeatedly if her yellow teeth could be fixed. I reassured her, but I moved on quickly—there was a line.

That night, I remembered her voice. There was a desperation in it. A cracking beneath the surface.
I wish I had paused. Asked her more. Told her something soothing.
Sometimes, it's not the words we say that stay with us.
It's the ones we didn't.

A Sentence That Became My Mantra

One old woman in a tattered shawl once placed her hand on mine and said, *"Beta, tum sab sun leti ho. Isi liye aaram milta hai."*

That line—that listening brings relief—echoes in me often.

On rushed days, when I'm falling behind on patients, or when I feel I'm not doing enough, I hear her voice.
And I slow down. I breathe. I listen.

Because care isn't just in what we do. It's in how we listen.

"Sometimes, a whisper says what a thousand words cannot."

And sometimes, that whisper changes the one listening forever.

11.

What I Saw in Their Silence

"Silence is not the absence of something.
It is the presence of everything."
— Gordon Hempton

There are stories that come through words—and then there are those that travel through silence.

Silence is not always empty. Sometimes it carries more weight than anything spoken.

In my journey through camps and clinics, I've often found myself listening to the pauses between words. The eyes that look away. The hands that fidget. The smiles that disappear too quickly.

Those were the moments that stayed with me. Because in those silent moments, I didn't just see patients. I saw truths.

And slowly, I began to understand: Silence was not a gap in the story. It was the story.

She walked in quietly, her saree edges frayed, her lips pressed into a thin line.

I asked gently, "Kya dikkat hai?"

She just nodded, sat down, and opened her mouth. Not a word.

Her molars were broken, gums swollen.

Still, she didn't speak.

I could see the stories she didn't tell—maybe shame, maybe fear, maybe just exhaustion.

As I examined her, she kept looking at the wall behind me.

That day, I realized silence can sit across from you like a person—breathing, shifting, waiting. And I learned to sit with it, without needing to fix it.

In one urban clinic, a man in a neatly ironed shirt came in for a routine check-up.
He had everything: insurance, time, even interest.

But he barely spoke.

He nodded, made polite gestures, but his silence wasn’t shyness. It was restraint—the kind people learn when they've been told emotions are weakness.

When I found signs of early-stage gum disease and explained the treatment, he nodded again. Still no words.

But just as he left, he paused, then turned and said quietly:

"Doctor, thank you for not making me feel dumb."

That one sentence said more than all the silence before it. And in that silence, I saw pride, fear, vulnerability—and gratitude.

Sometimes, children carry silence as armor.

One boy sat curled into the chair, holding his knees. His mother answered all my questions.
"Woh brush nahi karta. Kehne par bhi nahi."

When I looked at him and asked softly, "Tumhe kya lagta hai?" he didn’t reply.

But his eyes shimmered.

And in that moment, I realized he wasn't silent because he didn't care. He was silent because somewhere, someone had made him feel he wasn't allowed to speak.

I handed him a mirror and showed him how his teeth could be cleaned.

He didn't smile. But he took the mirror home.

That exchange stayed with me. Because in his silence, I saw generations of "children should be quiet" stitched into his soul.

In a camp in Sanjay Colony, a woman came for her daughter's check-up.

She stood behind, arms crossed, observing.

When I offered to check her too, she shook her head. "Main theek hoon," she said.

But she kept standing.

Watching.

I sensed a question behind her silence.

Finally, when her daughter was done, she asked, "Bachpan mein keede lage daant theek hote hain kya?"

I nodded, explained.

And she sat down.

Her silence hadn't been refusal.

It was testing.

Testing whether I was gentle enough. Patient enough. Human enough.

In her silence, I didn't see distance. I saw hope—hesitant, fragile hope.

The Sound of a Withheld Sob

In Kachchi Sarai, an older woman sat on the bench with her mouth open, jaw trembling.

Her teeth were loose. Some gone. She looked at me with eyes so tired, they seemed hollow.

She didn't speak.

But when I told her, gently, that she would need extractions and dentures, her hand slowly moved to cover her mouth.

And a tear slid down her cheek.

That tear spoke more than any case sheet ever could. It told me everything she didn't have the words for.

When Silence Became the Story

One day, I saw a young woman, beautifully dressed, makeup done with care.

She sat down, gave one-word answers, avoided mirrors.

Her teeth were fine. But her gums were bleeding.
I asked about stress.

She didn't answer.

Then, after a long pause, she said:

"Bas sab kuch sambhalna padta hai. Kabhi apne liye time hi nahi milta."

And that was all.

No drama. No breakdown.

Just one quiet confession.

And I understood: sometimes the silence is not about teeth. Sometimes it's about everything else that wears you down.

What I Learned in the Quiet

Silence has a posture.
Sometimes it slouches. Sometimes it folds its hands.
Sometimes it covers its mouth.
But always, it tells a story.

I've learned not to rush it. Not to fill it with instructions. Just to stay. And listen.

Some patients don't need solutions. They need space.

Some silences are asking,

"Will you judge me?" "Will you rush me?" "Will you really see me?"

And when you answer with gentleness, sometimes the silence lets go.

The Day Silence Changed Me

There was once a girl who came, sat down, and didn't say a word.

She let me examine her.

At the end, I asked if she had any questions.
She shook her head.
Then, right before leaving, she whispered,

"Mujhe laga aap bhi daantenge. Par aap toh... theek hain."

I smiled.

But something shifted in me that day.

Because silence isn't always fear. Sometimes it's a test of safety. And when someone finally speaks, it means you passed.

I used to think being a dentist was about treating teeth. Now I know it's also about reading quiet glances.

About the sigh before someone opens their mouth.

About the shrug that means more than a sentence.

What I saw in their silence wasn't absence. It was presence—of pain, of history, of resilience.

These silences became my greatest teachers. They made me softer. Slower. Wiser.
And most of all, they made me see:

That what remains unsaid often matters more than what is spoken.

*"Some of the loudest cries are silent.
Listen gently."*

Bridging The Gap

"Between what is said and what is heard, what is known and what is feared, there lies a space we often forget to explore: understanding."

Bridges aren't made of steel and stone alone. Sometimes, they are made of empathy. Of effort. Of listening more closely, even when no one is speaking.

This part of the book is about that space between two worlds: the world of the patient and the world of the provider. One is often soaked in silence, discomfort, myths, and hesitations. The other is lined with protocols, language, and systems. And in between lies the human experience.

Bridging the gap means learning how to meet patients not where we expect them to be, but where they are.

It means acknowledging that clinical knowledge is not enough—what's also needed is cultural sensitivity, emotional intelligence, and time. It means shifting from "treating" to "understanding." From fixing to listening. In the earlier sections of this book, I shared what I heard and saw—the voices, the silences, the readiness, the shame, the weight of delay. In this section, I shift the lens—not away from the patient, but toward the systems, perceptions, and relationships that influence care.

We will explore how distance isn't always geographical—it can also be emotional, generational, or linguistic. How access doesn't mean availability alone—it also means affordability, dignity, and clarity. And how change is possible, not when one side pulls harder, but when both sides walk toward each other.

These chapters are for everyone who has ever stood at the edge of that gap—uncertain whether to ask, to listen, to trust, or to care. And it is especially for those of us in the healthcare field who want to do more than treat symptoms—we want to see people.

Because dentistry, like all healing, happens not in isolation but in connection.

Let this part be a step toward that connection.

12.

The Fear Flies

"To truly heal someone, you must first understand what they fear."
— Dr. Rachel Naomi Remen

Sometimes, before a camp begins, I sit quietly with a cup of chai, watching people gather near the tent. Some come with folded forms. Some with folded worries. And some... just stand there—half a footstep away from the chair, fully engulfed in hesitation.

Fear doesn't always arrive with screams or sobs. Sometimes it enters the room wrapped in politeness. It sits with a polite smile, answers softly, and nods quickly—all while hoping the chair doesn't recline.

It hides in the pauses. In the shifting of feet. In the sudden dryness of the mouth.

I've seen fear wear many costumes—boldness, silence, jokes, anger, even complete denial.

And yet, it always speaks. Not in words, but in the spaces between them.

Fear in the Rural Camps

In a dusty little village called Basauli, I met an elderly woman who had walked over a kilometre to attend our camp.

"Bas dekh lijiye. Theek hoon," she said, as I gestured toward the chair.

Her fingers trembled. I offered her water. She refused. Her grip on the armrest was tighter than necessary. I began the examination slowly.

Halfway through, her eyes welled up.

"Pehli baar aayi hoon. Dar lagta hai. Kya nikaalenge daant?"
This wasn't just fear of pain. It was fear of loss. Of shame. Of not understanding what might happen next.

Fear doesn't just whisper.
Sometimes it stomps.

Sometimes it hides.
Sometimes it waits for us to look away.

Fear Dressed as Confidence

In Saviour Park, a polished society in Ghaziabad, a young professional walked in, phone in hand, power suit crisp.

"Quick cleaning. I have a meeting."

But as I put on gloves and reached for the scaler, she suddenly pulled her head back.

"Uh... wait. Is it going to bleed?"

I paused.

"Just a little discomfort. But we'll go slow."

And then, quietly, she admitted:

"I read something online... it said scaling makes teeth loose. I don't want gaps."

Behind the confidence was fear rooted in misinformation. In this case, Google, not a ghost, had spooked her.

The Boy Who Said Nothing

In a satellite clinic, a boy around Class 8 came with his mother. When I asked what the issue was, the mother said, *"Aap dekh lijiye."*

The boy wouldn't open his mouth.

When he finally did, I was shocked. A thick, stone-like layer of calculus covered every tooth—front, back, upper, lower. The teeth looked dressed in grey.

He mumbled he'd never brushed in his life.
I began scaling, but he resisted, flinching and muttering, *"Aap daant tod rahe ho."*

We managed to complete only a quarter. Four sittings were needed.

But he never came back.
I often wonder if shame had rooted deeper than the calculus. If fear of judgment kept him from ever returning.

Fear of Diagnosis

One of the most silent forms of fear is the fear of knowing.

Patients often delay visits not because they don't care, but because they care too much.

A woman once said:

"Main jaanti hoon kuch hoga. Par sunne se darr lagta hai."
That fear of confirmation—that something is wrong—can be stronger than the pain itself.

It's the same fear that stops people from opening test results, making calls, or looking in the mirror.

Inherited Fear

Some fears are not born from experience but passed down.

"Mummy kehti thi daant nikalna matlab aankhon pe asar padta hai."
"Dadaji kehte the brush se daant ghis jaate hain."

These aren't just myths. They're hand-me-down fears.

And they carry weight because they're wrapped in love and protection.

When we dismiss them as silly, we break trust.

Instead, I've learned to say:

"I understand why that worries you. But let me show you how it works now."

Because facts don't erase fear.

Understanding does.

Fear of Being Judged

Once, an elderly man sat in my chair. I asked how long he'd had the problem.

He hesitated, then said quietly, "*Zyada time ho gaya. Par dant dikhaane mein sharam aati thi. Gande hain.*"
His teeth were not even half as bad as his embarrassment.

Fear of being judged is powerful. And it doesn't discriminate. I've seen it in CEOs and housemaids alike.

In truth, people are not afraid of dentists.

They are afraid of shame. Afraid of being seen in their vulnerability. Afraid that their neglect makes them "less".

But what they need to hear is:

"You came today. That's what matters."

The Girl With the Brown Teeth

She came into the camp in Sultanpur with her sister.

"Mere daanton ki wajah se koi rishta nahi ho raha," she said softly.

Her teeth had fluorosis—deep brown stains and pits.
She wasn't in pain.
She was just tired.
Tired of rejection. Of smiles she didn't give. Of stares she had learned to absorb.

Her fear was different.
It wasn't fear of procedure.
It was fear that this was all she would ever be seen for.

We cleaned what we could, but more than her enamel, what needed healing was her self-worth.

Maybe she thought:

> Maybe they'll laugh. Maybe they'll say it can't be fixed.
Maybe they'll say nothing at all—which sometimes hurts more.

Sitting With Their Fears

Over the years, I've come to realize:
Fear is not a problem to fix. It's a presence to sit with.

When a patient hesitates, I no longer rush. When they say *"kal aayenge,"* I don't push.

Because sometimes, the bravest thing isn't sitting in the chair. It's deciding to walk toward it.
Just like the woman who once stood at the edge of the camp saying, *"She insisted I come along."*—fear rarely enters alone. It brings silence, questions, and sometimes... courage too.

"Fear is not always a barrier. Sometimes, it is just a waiting room where someone hopes they'll be understood."

And if we can sit with their fear—not as doctors, but as humans—we just might be the reason someone finally chooses to walk in.

13.

“Someone Told Me...” — Myths We Live By

"A myth is not a lie. It is a truth someone once believed, handed down without question."
— Anonymous

In a small village near Ghaziabad, under the shade of a neem tree, a woman in her seventies gently cupped my hand as I explained her treatment plan.

"Beta, aap daant mat saaf karo, woh hil jaayenge," she said, her voice full of caution, not defiance.

Her dupatta was faded, but neatly draped. Her eyes—clear, trusting, and worried—looked at me like I was too young to know better.

I smiled. Not because I found her words amusing, but because I had heard them many times before. From men in kurta-pyjamas, from working mothers in urban clinics, from college students in society camps.

Someone always says it: *"Scaling se daant hil jaate hain."*
And someone always means it.

Beliefs That Travel Generations

There is a moment in every dental camp where someone begins their story with: *"Someone told me..."*

Someone told them brushing too much will scrape the enamel. Someone told them removing a tooth would affect their vision. Someone told them sugar causes cavities but gud doesn't.

And they carry these stories like inherited songs—singing them to their children, rehearsing them before stepping into the clinic.

Like the young boy who refused to sit.

"Injection lagwaoge na toh haath kaam karna band ho jaata hai," he said, pressing into his mother.

I crouched beside him and smiled. *"Kisne bataya?"*

He looked away. *"Bhaiya ne. Unke friend ko hua tha."*

And just like that, a myth had traveled from a teenage rumor to a child's body.

The Whisper of Misinformation

In SCC heights—a gated society in Ghaziabad—a lady in crisp salwar came for a consultation but refused a scaling.

"Meri dost ne karwaya tha, baad mein daant hilne lage," she said with concern.

When I explained how tartar can act like cement, falsely holding teeth in place, she blinked. *"Then why didn't anyone tell us earlier?"*

It wasn't defiance. It was disappointment.
That myth wasn't her fault. It was the gap we left.

The Funny Ones—And the Dangerous Ones

A wrinkled grandfather once whispered, *"Doctor saab, daant nikalte waqt agar daant zameen pe gir gaya, toh daba ke mat jaaiyo. Warna dard kabhi nahi jaayega."* Another said, *"Chandi ka daant diabetes laata hai."*

And one school boy warned his friend, *"Neem ke tel se kida bhaag jaata hai, root canal ki zarurat nahi."*

We chuckle gently at these—but inside, we know the cost. Because while some myths are harmless, others delay treatment, deepen fear, and isolate patients.

Like the teenage girl who hid her teeth for years due to brown stains caused by fluorosis, told by her family that brushing harder would fix it. The stain remained. So did the shame.

Myth as Memory

"Why did you wait so long?"

They aren't just dental beliefs. They are reflections of a community's history with care. Or the lack of it..
In a camp at Duhai i, a man in his fifties showed off his yellow teeth with pride.

"Dekho, peele hain toh mazboot hain. Doctor ne bola strong enamel."

He thought yellow meant strong. He had learned to admire the color of damage.

In a satellite clinic, a boy barely in class 10 came with his mother. She said, *"Aap dekh lo."* He refused to open his mouth. When he did, it looked like his teeth were wearing stone jackets.

He had never brushed. Ever.

"Yeh sab toh dawai se theek ho jaayega na?" his mother asked, hopeful.
It took four visits to clean a quarter of his mouth. He never returned for the rest.

Shame.
Fear.
Silence.

Busting the Beliefs Gently

Sometimes I don't start with science. I start with a story.

"There was a man, just like you, who thought cleaning would loosen his teeth. But he trusted me, and today he can eat without pain."
Or I point to my own face: *"See my teeth? I get them cleaned too. Does it look like they're falling out?"*

Sometimes that lands better than a diagram.

Not Lies, But Incomplete Truths

The biggest myths are rarely random. They often come from a half-understood truth.

Scaling loosens teeth — because disease was hidden beneath tartar.

Charcoal toothpaste is best — because it's natural, but too abrasive.

Tooth extraction causes blindness — rooted in fear, not anatomy.

Milk teeth don't matter — until they cause infections that hurt.

What Breaks a Myth?

Not arguments. Moments.

Like when a woman's pain finally wins over her inherited fears. Like when a child giggles after the procedure that didn't hurt. Like when a man walks in hiding his mouth and leaves smiling.

These are the new stories. The ones that replace old ones.

"Someone Told Me..."

Those three words don't irritate me anymore.
They humble me.

Because if someone told them something untrue, maybe I can be someone too. Someone who replaces fear with clarity.

Not by dismissing. But by listening.

Not by laughing. But by honoring the story they carry—and offering a better one in return.

"Sometimes, what heals isn't truth alone.
It's how gently it is offered."

14.

What They Thought vs. What Was True

"Fear has many voices, but truth needs only one moment to be heard."
– L.R. Knost

The camp had just begun. The sun was still stretching its arms, rising above the rooftops of Sanjay Colony. Volunteers were unpacking tables, sterilizers, pamphlets. And patients… were arriving with quiet expectations and noisy fears.

There is a silence that settles before the first question is asked.

It's in the eyes of the patient. The grip on the armrest. The hesitation in their step.

They think they know what they're about to walk into.

They think it's going to hurt. Be expensive. Be shameful. They think they'll be judged.

And then something shifts.

Sometimes, it's a smile. Sometimes, it's a conversation. Sometimes, it's the kindness in how we say, *"You're not too late."*

The Boy Who Thought He Would Be Scolded

In a dusty lane of Sanjay Colony, a boy barely in class seven came with his grandmother. He had a decayed molar that had blackened, broken, and become painful enough to keep him awake at night.

I greeted him gently, but he didn't respond. His eyes were down. When I asked him to sit, he hesitated.

His grandmother whispered, *"Doctor se darte hain. Pehli baar aaye hain."*

As he sat, I noticed his hands clenched tight around the edges of the chair. I began speaking softly.
"You know, my first patient today was even more scared than you. But he left laughing."

He glanced up—just a little.

As I examined him, he flinched.
"Does it hurt?" He shook his head.

"Then what are you thinking?" He paused.

"Agar daant zyada kharab ho gaya hoga toh aap daant hi nikaal doge... bina bataye."

There it was.

Not fear of pain. Not fear of tools.

Fear of being out of control. Fear of being shamed.

"We'll do nothing without telling you first," I said. "You're part of this too."

He nodded, finally. And the hand that had gripped the chair? It relaxed.

I've come to believe that fear is rarely loud. Most times, it tiptoes in quietly—hidden behind practiced smiles, folded arms, and a hundred rehearsed reasons for delay.

The Man from Raj Nagar

At an urban location camp setup in Raj Nagar, a man in his 50s came in, his shirt tucked, leather folder in hand. He seemed confident. But as soon as I asked about the problem, his words tumbled.

"Doctor, I know I should've come earlier. But I thought it'd be too costly. I thought... it'd be embarrassing."

I nodded. *"You're not alone."*

He looked at me.

"You see this?" he pointed at his front teeth, slightly yellowed, uneven.

"I stopped smiling in meetings. Because someone once joked. I laughed along—but it stayed."

And just like that, we weren't talking about teeth anymore.

We were talking about self-worth.

He had assumed dentists only focused on cosmetic perfection. That we measured people by the whiteness of their teeth.
But that day, he walked away not just with a treatment plan—but with his dignity intact.

Because truth, when offered gently, doesn't just inform. It restores.

The Eyebrow Confusion

A young man once asked, *"Scaling karwa liya toh kya mujhe roz karwana padega? Jaisa eyebrows hota hai?"*
We both laughed. *"Teeth aren't eyebrows,"* I said. *"And no, you won't need monthly appointments—just good habits."*
That laughter made room for truth to land gently.

What Patients Often Think...

"They'll judge me for not brushing enough."

"It'll cost too much, and they'll suggest things I can't afford."

"It'll be painful. I've heard horror stories."
"I'll be scolded."
These thoughts are rarely spoken aloud. But I see them. In the delay. The crossed arms. The reluctance to make eye contact.

And What They Discover Instead

That pain can be managed with kindness.

That care doesn't have to be unaffordable.

That we explain everything before we act.
That they are not alone in their delay.

One woman in a rural camp told me:

"Main soch rahi thi daanto mein keeda hoga, aur aap log daant nikaal doge bina puchhe. Lekin aapne toh pyaar se bataya, dikhaya bhi."

She came expecting a battle.
She left with trust.

The Elderly Woman Who Took Pride in Pain

In one of our camps, a frail woman arrived with two others supporting her. She had a yellow card in her hand—the kind given during free treatment camps. Her hands trembled. Her back was bent.

She said, proudly, *"Mere daant saare hain, aur kabhi kharab nahi hue."*

But when she opened her mouth, I was stunned.

Her teeth were intact, yes. But they were held by almost nothing.
The gums had receded. The bone had dissolved.

I could have removed any of her teeth with two fingers.

But she was proud. Because she had been told that chewing tobacco keeps teeth strong.

It hadn't.

It had robbed her of nourishment, and over time, her health.

But I didn't shatter that pride in one moment. I respected it. Then gently, slowly, I told her what was really happening.

That truth didn't come as a blow. It arrived like light slipping through the cracks.

The Girl with Stains

In Sultanpur, a girl sat quietly behind her sister.
She had visible brown stains on her front teeth—likely fluorosis. She kept looking down.

Her mother spoke for her. *"Shaadi mein dikkat aa rahi hai. Ladke ke ghar se mana aa gaya."*

I asked the girl to speak. She hesitated, then softly said:

"Main zyada nahi bolti. Log muh ki taraf dekhte hain."

She thought her stains were a punishment. She thought she'd always be rejected.

She didn't know it could be managed, improved, even polished.

Her silence said, *"I don't deserve better."*

Our words said otherwise.

Truth Doesn't Always Arrive with Data

Sometimes I want to explain everything:
That calculus can hold in teeth falsely. That scaling doesn't loosen teeth, it saves them. That pain is manageable. That judgement has no place here.

But then I pause. Because sometimes, it's not facts people need first.

It's warmth.

It's the comfort of someone looking at them not with clinical precision—but with human care.

Beyond Assumptions

They thought it would hurt. They thought it would cost too much. They thought they would be scolded, humiliated. They thought it was too late.

They were wrong.
And thank God for that.

Because when truth finally met them, it wasn't harsh. It was healing.

A Mirror for Ourselves Too

We, too, carry assumptions.

We assume patients don't care. Or that they're careless. We assume they don't value their health.

But when I sat with them, listened, looked—I saw it:

They cared deeply. They were scared. They were misinformed. They were overwhelmed.

They wanted help. They just didn't know how to ask..

The Moment of Reconciliation

I remember an elderly man once stood up after a consultation, and with tears in his eyes said:

"Aap log alag hain. Maine socha tha doctor daantega. Aap toh samjhe."

And I wanted to say:

We are not different. We are just trying to return you to the truth you forgot: that you matter.

Closing the Gap

This chapter isn't just about what patients thought. It's about what we assumed too.
It's about the space between fear and healing. And the bridge we build, one gentle truth at a time.

Because sometimes, all it takes to rewrite a fear is one sentence, one touch, one human moment that says—you are safe now.

"Fear has many voices, but truth needs only one moment to be heard."

15.

Bridges, Not Barriers

"The goal is not to fix people. The goal is to walk beside them as they remember they were never broken." – Unknown

She stood near the edge of the camp, under the shade of a neem tree, eyes flitting from the banner to the crowd to the folding chairs. She wasn't holding a form. Her hands were tucked into the ends of her dupatta.

"Aaj free check-up hai na?" she asked softly.

I nodded.

She didn't sit immediately. She walked a slow circle around the mobile van, watching. Listening. Carrying something unspoken.

Twenty minutes later, she sat down. Not because her pain had worsened—but because something inside her had softened. That first step, that quiet act of sitting,

became a bridge. From doubt to trust. From silence to story.
This chapter is about that bridge.

Listening as the First Step

We often look for answers in policy, in outreach, in awareness drives. But over time, I've realized that real change begins with something quieter: listening.

In a rural camp in Guldhar, a man asked, *"Daant nikalne mein kitna waqt lagta hai?"* He didn't sit. He didn't register. He just wanted to know. That was his first step. And in his question, I heard both fear and curiosity.

He didn't need a lecture.

He needed clarity. A gentle one.

Information is a bridge. But only when it's offered with patience, not pressure.

When we speak, we share knowledge.

When we listen, we create connection.

The Language of Care

One thing I've learned: words matter. They can either build a wall or lay the first plank of a bridge.

Saying, builds a barrier.

Saying, *"You're here now. That matters,"* builds a bridge.

I no longer say *"scaling."* I say, *"We'll clean gently, so your teeth feel lighter."* Instead of, *"You've neglected your oral health,"* I say, *"You've carried a lot. Let's take care of this together."*

That's not sugarcoating. That's translation.

Care must be spoken in the language of comfort.

Designing for Dignity

I dream of a clinic with sunlight. With chairs that don't creak, and walls that don't make patients feel like they're in trouble.

I dream of a place where the first question isn't, *"What's your problem?"* but *"How are you feeling today?"* Because dignity is not decoration. It's design.

Patients shouldn't feel like cases. They should feel like guests.

Imagine waiting rooms with warm light, not harsh tubes. Posters drawn by children, not diagrams of bleeding gums. A space where fear can sit down and breathe.

Healing starts long before the probe enters the mouth. It starts when someone feels welcomed.

From Outreach to Inreach

We often measure impact by how far our outreach spreads.

But what if we also practiced inreach?
Not just reaching villages or gated communities. But reaching hearts. Early. Quietly.

In schools, we teach brushing techniques. What if we also taught children not to fear dentists?

In families, we teach kids to say *"Namaste"* to elders.
What if we also taught them to say, *"Mujhe dard ho raha hai"* without shame?
Fear grows in the absence of familiarity.

Trust grows in repetition. In softness.

When a Bench Becomes a Bridge

At a camp in a village of Muradnagar, a girl sat on a wooden bench beneath a mulberry tree. She didn't speak. Her dupatta covered half her face. Others came and went. She stayed.
Then, after an hour, she whispered, *"Bas dekh lijiye ek baar."*

We checked. Fluorosis. Brown patches on her front teeth.
"Shaadi nahi ho rahi," she said, voice flat.

We talked. About treatment. About hope.

She didn't ask for a solution. She asked to be seen.
That bench wasn't just wood. It was a bridge. Between shame and courage. Between hiding and healing.

Clinics must carry that bench within them. That spirit of slowness, of safety.

A Clinic That Walks

Not everyone can walk into a clinic. So sometimes, the clinic must walk.

It must walk into temples, schools, parks.

It must sit under trees. Wait without hurrying. Listen without interrupting.

Because care isn't a destination.

It's a presence.

At a camp in Raj Nagar, a man in a crisp shirt circled the mobile van three times. Then finally said, *"Bas consult karna hai."*

He hadn't seen a dentist in over ten years.
"Kaam mein busy tha," he said.

But when we began the check-up, he exhaled.

"Didn't realize how tense I was," he admitted.

Tension doesn't always announce itself. It hides behind routines. But the moment someone sits—and sighs—a bridge has been crossed.

Community as Care

In Khera, five women sat under a mango tree, passing a steel tiffin. Joking about their teeth. Laughing softly.

But when it was time to get checked, they fell silent.

"Main pehle jaaungi. Agar theek laga, toh tum log bhi aana," one said.

She became the bridge for the others.

Healing can begin in circles. In shared courage.
When women walk in groups, care feels less frightening.
Sometimes, community is the clinic.

The Invisible Bridges

There are bridges we don't see.

A mother translating symptoms for her silent daughter.

A boy bringing his grandmother because she's scared to come alone.

A patient removing all their jewelry before treatment, saying, *"Doctorji, yeh ladayi ke liye tayyari hai."*

These small gestures are acts of preparation, of bravery.

Not everyone will say, *"I'm scared."*

Some will just stand nearby, holding space for their own fear.

We must learn to notice these bridges. And walk toward them.

The Future We Can Build

A future where oral health isn't a luxury.
Where girls aren't rejected for stains they were born with.

Where patients aren’t told to be strong—but are told, *"Take your time."*
Where clinics smell like care, not chemicals.

Where dentists listen first. Probe later.

Where pain is not minimized.

Where silence is understood.
Where every patient is met not with assumptions, but with curiosity.

My Bridge

This book was not meant to preach. It was meant to pause.

To say: I see you.

Whether you're a patient who has waited too long.

Or a caregiver who wants to do better.

This is not a manual.

It’s a mirror.

Of what we've ignored. Of what we can now choose to change.

We don't need to fix everything overnight.
We just need to start walking.
And build bridges.

One kind word at a time. One story at a time. One hand reaching out—without judgment.

Because healing doesn't always arrive with instruments.

Sometimes, it arrives in a sentence:

"Aayiye, baithiye. Hum dheere karenge."

Bridges don't erase fear. They offer a way across it.
And maybe that's what we all need.
Not to be told it won't hurt.

But to be reminded:

You won't go through it alone.

Beyond The Mouth

"Not everything that is faced can be changed, but nothing can be changed until it is faced."
— James Baldwin

We are trained to look at the mouth—to examine gums, check occlusion, diagnose decay. But the more time I spent with patients, the more I realized: the real stories don't always sit inside the mouth.

They live behind the eyes. In the pause before a sentence. In what a patient doesn't say, even after being asked twice.

Pain is rarely just physical. A toothache may begin in the mouth—but it often carries the weight of exhaustion, loneliness, anxiety, or quiet shame. And over time, I learned that when someone says, *"It hurts here,"* what they might truly mean is, *"I'm carrying too much, and I don't know where else it can go."*

This part of the book is about those layers.

It explores what oral health can reveal about a person's life—but more importantly, what it cannot hide. It reflects on how stress wears down enamel, how trauma clenches jaws, how depression forgets to brush, and how silence keeps even the most urgent questions unspoken.

It's not about teeth alone. It is about the emotional body that enters quietly with every patient—their burdens, beliefs, and untold truths.

It's also about us—as caregivers, as dentists, as humans. What do we carry into the room? How do our words land? Can we see beyond the swelling and ask the questions that matter?

The chapters ahead are not just case studies. They are confessions, revelations, and quiet revolutions. They remind us that true care doesn't end with a diagnosis.

It begins where the chart ends.

Beyond the checklist.
Beyond the clinic.
Beyond the mouth.

16.

Healing On Both Sides

"A delay is not a denial. It is often a quiet plea for understanding."

There is a moment in every journey where research and reflection meet reality.

Mine arrived in the form of a number.

93.4%

That's how many participants in my study delayed dental care.

Some delayed because of fear. Others because of cost. Many because they believed, *"It's not serious enough."*

But behind each reason, I saw something deeper: procrastination rooted in pain.

Not just the pain of a toothache, but the ache of anxiety. The tightness of stress. The silent scream of stigma. I remember sitting at my desk, reviewing responses—line after line of reasons, hesitations, avoidance patterns. It didn't feel like data. It felt like confession.
When I began this research, I thought I was studying behaviour. In truth, I was studying coping.

Dental attendance, I discovered, is less about health and more about readiness—readiness to confront discomfort, to prioritize oneself, to trust a system that has often ignored deeper fears.
Readiness is psychological, emotional, social. It is built slowly, painfully, through education, empathy, and repeated reassurance.

A person doesn't skip a dental visit simply because they're lazy. They skip it because they're scared. Because they're overwhelmed. Because they've never been told their pain matters before it becomes unbearable.

This is where dental science must evolve. Not only in tools or techniques—but in understanding why people delay.

And the answer, over and over, is this: they don't feel safe enough to show up.

Let's pause here.

Consider the 51% of participants who had moderate dental anxiety. The 35.3% who had severe anxiety. The 31% with high levels of procrastination. Now overlay this with the 93.4% delay in dental care.

The picture is clear: the burden isn't just clinical. It's emotional.

This is where the bridge must be built—not just from the clinic to the community, but from fear to familiarity, from stigma to support.

This book, at its heart, is that bridge.

Between clinics and communities. Between hesitation and healing. Between silence and seeking help.
The data from my research gave me charts, tables, and correlation coefficients. One finding struck me deeply: participants with better oral health and regular visits had lower anxiety and procrastination.

Another: the strongest reason for delay was the belief that a dental visit isn't necessary without acute symptoms.
That's not just a misunderstanding—it's a systemic failure in education and communication. We've normalized suffering until it screams.

But what I remember most aren't the charts.

I remember the eyes.

Eyes that flickered with hesitation. Eyes that widened with relief. Eyes that blinked back tears when someone finally said, *"You're not too late."*

I've watched patients apologize for delaying treatment—as if delay was a moral failure.

I've listened to women whisper that they hid their swelling to avoid judgment from their in-laws.

I've seen men pretend stoicism, only to ask quietly, *"Will this hurt too much? I have to get back to work."*

Delay is not weakness. It is a symptom. Of fear. Of systems that silence. Of a culture that often punishes sensitivity.

My final message is not a conclusion. It is an invitation.

To every caregiver: Look beyond the mouth. Hear the hesitation. Honour it. Let your first tool be listening.

To every patient: You are not weak for waiting. You are brave for showing up. You are not late—you are right on time.

To the policymakers: Prevention is not a luxury. It is a lifeline. Fund it, normalize it, decentralize it.

To the next generation: Don't just build taller chairs. Build longer benches.
We live in a world that often punishes delay.

We expect efficiency, promptness, initiative. But healing does not operate on a schedule. It blooms in the soil of trust.

And while 93.4% may be a statistic, it is also a mirror. It reflects what we've missed—but also what we can mend.

Let us mend it by softening our approach. By noticing the patient who walks in and says nothing. By respecting the silence. By honoring the courage that finally overcame hesitation.

If we listen. If we soften. If we stay.

Because behind every mouthful of silence lies a heartful of hope.

And sometimes, that hope begins with a whisper:

"Aayiye, baithiye. Ab der nahi hui."

This is not just a book about dentistry. It is a call to tenderness. A call to slow down and truly see the people who come to us—not just as patients, but as people seeking permission to heal.

And to them, I say:

You are welcome.
You are worthy.
You are never too late.

17.

Transforming the Chair – A Guide for Healthcare Providers

"Compassion is not an add-on. It's a clinical tool."

When a patient walks into a dental setting, they don't just carry symptoms. They carry silence. And that silence often began long before they entered the clinic.

As healthcare providers, we are trained to diagnose, to treat, to restore. But rarely are we taught to pause. To sit with fear before we sit with files. To address the emotional cavity before we reach the oral one.

It's time we transformed how we practice—not with more tools, but with more trust.

The CARE Framework
A model designed to embed empathy and behavior-awareness into everyday dental care:

STEPS	ACTION	OUTCOME
C	Communicate before treating	Reduces perceived threat
A	Acknowledge anxiety	Builds emotional safety
R	Reduce stigma	Preserves dignity
E	Engage through empathy	Builds trust, improves compliance

What You Can Do – Today, Not Someday

1. Change the Tone Before the Tool

• Start every first-time consult with a question like: "What's been stopping you from coming earlier?"
• Avoid technical jargon until rapport is built. Replace "RCT needed" with "We'll gently clean the infection to stop the pain."

2. Empathy Training Isn't Optional

• Propose in-clinic weekly role-play sessions among interns and staff.
• Incorporate mirror exercises: Have providers sit in the patient's chair while another simulates a stressful conversation.

A 2021 pilot study in Mumbai showed that interns trained in reflective listening improved patient follow-up by 19%.

Field Insight: What Made One Camp Different

In a dental camp in Muradnagar, a volunteer sat with patients in the waiting area—not to register, but to talk. She asked simple things: "Have you ever had a painful experience before?" or "What are you worried about today?"

That alone led to a 27% increase in patients opting for on-site procedures instead of referrals.

Reframing "Difficult Patients"

Many times, we label patients as "non-compliant" or "irregular." But what if we rephrased them as "emotionally unequipped" or "unready yet"? Our role isn't to push readiness. It's to create a space where readiness feels safe.

Small Changes, Big Impact – In Clinics

Traditional Approach	Transformed Approach
"Open your mouth."	"Take your time. Let me know when you're ready."
Token-based calling	Name-based welcoming ("Hello, Ms. Sharma, please come in.")
Quick documentation	Brief pre-counsel chat: "How are you feeling today?"
Prioritising patients	Prioritising comfort

An Implementation Blueprint: The "Comfort Protocol"

Every dental department or private clinic can initiate a Comfort Protocol using:

1. Training Modules (once/month): On trauma-informed care, emotional first aid
2. Patient Feedback Cards: With prompts like "Did you feel heard?"
3. Staff Incentives: Reward soft-skill excellence (not just speed or technical accuracy)

Strategy at the Chairside

As someone preparing for a career in healthcare consulting, I see this now with a double vision:

- Clinician: Each patient is a person with history, hesitation, and hope.
- Consultant: Each hesitation is a data point. A bottleneck. A fixable moment.

To fix systems, we must first honor stories.
What if we saw every dental chair not as a station for treatment, but as a space of transformation? Where the real procedure is not just physical—but emotional readiness.
Where silence isn't rushed, but respected.
Where showing up is seen as courage—not delay.

Because healing starts before the drill.

It starts the moment we say: "I'm glad you came."

18.

Policy That Listens – Recommendations for Policymakers

True public health policy doesn't begin in boardrooms. It begins in doorways—of homes, of clinics, of hesitation.

While my research revealed emotional and behavioral gaps, it also pointed to structural silences—places where systems were absent or insufficient. For policymakers, the challenge is not just creating new policies, but listening closely enough to shape the ones that matter.

The 3A Policy Lens: AWARENESS, ACCESS, AFFORDABILITY

A framework to build targeted, high-impact oral health policy.

Pillar	Policy Intervention	Expected Outcome

Awareness	Mass campaigns in schools, ASHA training, oral health radio jingles	Increased early intervention
Access	Mobile dental vans in rural areas, school screenings, satellite OPDs	Geographic coverage expands
Affordability	Subsidized routine check-ups, preventive care incentivesReduced long-term system burden	Embedding Oral Health in Preventive Ecosystems

- Add a mandatory oral health module in school health programs.
- Train community health workers to deliver oral screenings during routine house visits.
- Include dental anxiety detection as part of adolescent health initiatives.
- Incentivize village health committees that track oral health visits per household.

Case Insight: What a "Free Dental Check-up" Campaign Missed

In a district in UP, a week-long free dental camp saw low turnout despite heavy promotion. Interviews revealed fear and confusion: people thought 'free' meant experimental, or were unaware of the services offered.

A better-designed campaign would have included storytelling ads, pre-camp emotional counseling, and community leaders as health ambassadors.

Policy Blueprint: What to Build in the Next 5 Years

1. Dental care coverage under Ayushman Bharat for preventive services, not just extractions.
2. Oral health reporting indicators in district-level health data dashboards.
3. Public-private partnerships with NGOs for emotional literacy in oral care.
4. Special grant for behavioral health research in dental institutes.

The problem of delayed dental care is not just psychological—it's structural. By embedding awareness, access, and affordability into public health policy, we move from reacting to dental disease to preventing it.

And that shift—from cure to care—is what true policymaking looks like.

19.

Beyond the Family Gate – Empowering Patients & Communities

Behind every delayed visit is a family, a neighbor, a whispered myth. Empowering patients doesn't begin with instruction—it begins with inclusion. If we want to reduce silent suffering, we must turn passive observers into active participants.

This chapter is about how community-level strategies—rooted in trust, cultural intelligence, and shared accountability—can shift oral health behavior from reaction to prevention.

The "RIPPLE MODEL" of Health Dialogue

Information alone doesn't change behavior. Trust does.

LAYER	WHO	ROLE
Core	Patient	Receives care, shares fear

Immediate Circle	Family/Friends	Influence health-seeking action
Community Ring	Local leaders, teachers, shopkeepers	Normalize check-ups
Outer Network	NGOs, digital platforms	Amplify dialogue, fight myths

Patient Education is Not a Poster – It's a Process

- Host oral health storytelling circles in anganwadis and schools.
- Encourage 'Dental Day' in families—once a year check-ins done together.
- Develop myth-busting WhatsApp video snippets in local dialects.
- Use marriage bureaus, SHGs, and women's collectives as oral health ambassadors.

Community Innovation: The "DENTAL DIDI" Model

Inspired by the ASHA worker model, 'Dental Didis' are trained local women who:

• Identify dental anxiety cases in their area
• Provide emotional first aid and basic hygiene education
• Assist camps and link patients to dental vans

Why Collective Action Works

We respond faster to what feels familiar and endorsed. When families and local networks become oral health allies, check-ups become rituals—not reactions.

Think of it this way:
• If one person checks their mouth, they remember.
• If five people do it together, they remind each other.
• If a whole village does it during Dental Week, it becomes a norm.

Healthcare doesn't happen in isolation. It happens in tea stalls, group chats, schoolyards, kitchens. Empowering communities to take ownership of dental health creates ripple effects of change.

Because the greatest agent of transformation isn't always the dentist.

Sometimes, it's a sister.

A neighbor.

A nudge.

20.

Digital Bridges – Where Technology Meets Humanity

In the quiet spaces between pain and care lies a powerful tool—technology. But technology alone doesn't solve emotional barriers. It enables solutions when guided by empathy.

This chapter explores how digital interventions can serve as bridges—not replacements—for trust-building in oral healthcare. When used mindfully, tech can make the first step toward care feel less daunting, more human.

The Tele-Trust Chain – A Patient-Centric Digital Pathway

A multi-step digital model that supports patients through anxiety, access, and action:

	STEPS	FUNCTIONS

Step 1	Symptom Checker	Patient inputs symptoms via chatbot in their regional language
Step 2	Anxiety Score	Uses MDAS-based prompts to flag dental anxiety
Step 3	Counseling Video	Shows 1-minute stories from real patients
Step 4	Clinic Connector	Suggests nearest certified low-cost centers

WhatsApp Nudges – Microcommunication, Major Impact

A series of regional-language WhatsApp messages sent over two weeks post-camp increased follow-up rates by 35% in pilot zones. These messages didn't just remind—they reassured.

Sample messages:

• "You've already taken the bravest step—showing up."

• "Your smile matters. We're here when you're ready."

Tone, frequency, and familiarity make all the difference.
Designing Digital for Emotion, Not Just Efficiency

- Use patient names and familiar visuals in app UIs.
- Replace error messages with calming prompts ("It's okay to try again.")
- Allow one-tap "talk to someone" buttons in symptom checkers.
- Build feedback loops to track not just usage—but comfort.

Future Vision: A National Oral Health App

Envision a low-bandwidth, multi-lingual platform integrated with:

- Symptom-to-care journey (tele-triage to in-person)
- Digital dental card for treatment history
- Emotional readiness self-assessments
- Push notifications for preventive dental education

This isn't just about digitizing health—it's about humanizing digital.

In the gap between knowing you need help and asking for it, digital tools can hold a patient's hand—quietly, gently, effectively. But only when built with care.

Because true health-tech doesn't just connect clinics to people. It connects people to their courage.

21.

Designing Dignity – The Role of Clinic Spaces

"Architecture can heal. Or it can harden."

The way a clinic is designed—the sounds, the seats, the words on the wall—shapes how a patient feels long before treatment begins.

This chapter explores how even low-cost physical and emotional design changes in dental clinics and camps can foster trust, safety, and dignity.

Emotional Architecture – Mapping the Patient Journey

Think beyond logistics. Think feelings. Each point in a clinic's flow has an emotional impact:

TOUCH POINT	EMOTION TRIGGERE D	DESIGN CUE
Entrance	Apprehension	Welcome sign with soft lighting and a calming quote
Waiting Area	Anxiety builds	Soft seating, plants, calming visuals
Reception	Risk of judgment	Greet by name, offer water, smile
Consultation	Vulnerability	Doctor sits at eye level, uses pauses to listen
Exit	Relief or confusion	Clear written next steps, a thank-you card or note

Design Interventions That Heal

Replace hard metal benches with warm-toned, cushioned seats where possible.

Use posters showing patient stories—not just technical dental charts.

Create privacy zones using foldable screens or curtains in crowded settings.

Avoid loud token number systems. Use name-based or digital visual callouts.

Add calming music or nature sounds in background—especially in waiting areas.

The "Message Wall" - Words That Uplift

In one clinic, we added a blank board titled:

> *"What helped me show up today..."*

Patients wrote:

"My daughter said I deserved this."

"I was scared, but the nurse smiled first."

"I waited 3 years. I'm proud I came."

These notes became mirrors of courage—reflecting strength to the next patient in line.

From Clinics to Camps - Dignity Travels Too

Even temporary field camps can become spaces of care and comfort:

Set up shaded waiting areas with mats or chairs.

Appoint greeters—not just registration clerks—who explain what's happening.

Use printed or visual boards to guide patients through the station flow.

Offer takeaway cards with follow-up details and kind messages like: *"Thank you for trusting us today. You matte*r."

Conclusion

Healthcare doesn't begin with a diagnosis.
It begins the moment someone crosses a threshold—physical or emotional.

By designing for dignity, we make that threshold easier to cross.

Because a chair can be metal or memory.
Let's choose memory—the kind that reminds patients:

You were seen. You mattered. You were safe.

Ground Realities - Voices From The Field

The following section presents raw insights, stories, and data collected during this study. These voices form the foundation of the frameworks presented earlier

The Data Speaks

"Quantifying the Silence"

In healthcare, data is not just a series of numbers—it is a mirror reflecting silent struggles, hidden fears, and missed opportunities. This chapter draws heavily from a structured research study I conducted among approximately 300 participants in Muradnagar, India, later published in the Asian Journal of Dental Sciences (2024). By blending field observations with validated psychometric tools, this study quantifies the silent delays that often go unnoticed until it is too late.

Key Findings at a Glance

The research revealed startling patterns in patient behavior:

- 93.4% of participants admitted to delaying dental treatment.
- Only 7.3% reported visiting a dentist regularly once or twice a year.
- 35.3% exhibited high levels of dental anxiety.

- 55% reported moderate stress; 23% reported high stress levels.
- 31% demonstrated high procrastination tendencies.

Delay was most strongly associated with the belief that treatment is not necessary unless pain becomes unbearable.

Understanding the Silence

The reasons for delay were not purely logistical. Emotional and psychological barriers played a central role:

- Fear of pain or bad experiences.
- Denial of seriousness until symptoms worsen.
- High treatment cost concerns.
- Cultural stigma associated with showing weakness.
- Lack of perceived urgency or awareness.

The dominant emotional driver was *DENIAL*: patients acknowledged symptoms but underestimated their significance until serious deterioration occurred.

Behavioral Patterns by Demographic Group

A deeper demographic breakdown revealed:

- Females reported higher levels of procrastination and anxiety compared to males.
- Socio-economic background influenced the likelihood of seeking preventive care.
- Psychological stress was notably higher among working-age individuals (25–40 years).

The Socio-Economic Divide

Most participants belonged to the lower middle and upper middle classes, highlighting that even economically stable individuals experience significant behavioral barriers to seeking timely care.

What the Data Means for Us

These insights are not just academic—they have direct implications for hea**lthcare providers, policymakers, and communities:**

For Healthcare Providers:

Training in empathy, communication, and soft counseling is vital to overcoming patient fear and denial.

For Policymakers:

Accessibility improvements alone are not enough. Behavioral education and mass communication efforts are critical.

For Families and Individuals:

Normalizing preventive care conversations within families can break the cycle of avoidance and silence.

The numbers speak volumes.
And if we listen carefully, they reveal not only hidden pain, but also pathways to systemic healing.

What Lies Beneath

"Patient Psychology and Behavioral Barriers"

During fieldwork, I met patients who hid pain behind a smile, who dismissed their bleeding gums as *"nothing serious,"* and who genuinely believed that no visit was needed until their teeth *"hurt badly."*

Real Voices:

"I didn't think bleeding gums were serious."
"I'll only go when the pain is unbearable."
"I'm afraid of what they'll find, and how they'll judge me."

Behavioral Observations:

Denial & Shame: Many patients avoided care not due to ignorance, but because of social shame or fear of judgment. Some even believed dental issues were self-inflicted and thus shameful.

Fear Conditioning: Prior traumatic experiences with dental care led to avoidance behavior. Memories of pain, unfriendly doctors, or expensive procedures shaped negative attitudes.

Health Belief Model in Practice: Patients perceived low susceptibility unless visible symptoms occurred, underestimating preventive care. They lacked awareness of asymptomatic diseases like periodontitis.

Learned Helplessness: Chronic neglect of oral health led to resignation. Patients felt that oral problems were a normal part of life and nothing could truly help them.

Cultural Narratives: In many communities, dental care is considered non-essential unless critical. Dental pain is often treated with home remedies until unbearable.

Psychological Impact: Avoidance behavior contributes to heightened anxiety, low health literacy, and a vicious cycle of neglect. Understanding these psychological patterns is essential for developing interventions that inspire behavioral change, not just awareness.

Bridging the System

"Solutions for a Silent Crisis"

Breaking the silence in oral healthcare requires more than surface-level fixes. It demands a systemic redesign that integrates accessibility, trust, education, innovation, and empathy. Below is a structured framework to help organize impactful interventions—applicable across policy, technology, families, and clinics.

The solutions proposed in this chapter are grounded not just in personal interactions but also validated through structured primary research. The patterns, behaviors, and gaps identified were rigorously studied and peer-reviewed, providing a strong foundation for system-level recommendations.

Introducing the B.R.I.D.G.E. Model

To address the complexity of patient delay and silence, I propose the B.R.I.D.G.E. Model—a strategic, actionable framework to drive change in oral healthcare:

B – Behavioral Support (Training for providers, counseling)
R – Reinforcement through Community Campaigns
I – Innovation via Technology & Telehealth
D – Dialogue with Families and Peer Support
G – Government Policy & Education Integration
E – Empathy-Driven Clinical Design
Each pillar targets both systemic gaps and human behavior.

Access & Outreach
How It Helps: Increases visibility and reduces distance—literally and psychologically—between patients and care.

Emotional Engagement & Trust
How It Helps: Patients fear judgment more than pain. Rebuilding trust requires safe spaces, empathetic language, and visible support.

Policy & Public Education
How It Helps: Education doesn't change behavior unless it's repeated, relatable, and reinforced through culture.

Innovation & Technology
How It Helps: Tech lowers access barriers and boosts consistency. It personalizes care while maintaining scale.

Empathy in Practice (Clinic Design + Staff Behavior)
How It Helps: A gentle, non-clinical experience can significantly reduce anxiety and promote return visits.

Closing Reflection

Silence in oral healthcare is not accidental—it is learned, passed down, and socially reinforced. But so is change. By creating systems that are empathetic, innovative, structured, and human-first, we can build a healthcare model that listens before it prescribes, educates before it judges, and prevents before it treats.

Potential Impact of Bridging the Silence

If the behavioral and systemic barriers to timely dental care are addressed through the solutions proposed, the broader impact could include:

Reduction in Advanced Dental Treatments:

Early intervention can reduce the need for costly procedures like extractions, root canals, and prosthetics by up to 40–50%.

Healthcare Cost Savings:

Preventive dental care costs 4 to 10 times less than emergency or rehabilitative treatments, easing the financial burden on both individuals and public health systems.

Workplace Productivity Gains:

Fewer dental emergencies mean reduced absenteeism. Studies show that untreated dental issues contribute to significant workday losses annually.

Mental Health Improvement:

Timely dental care reduces chronic pain, improves self-esteem, and lowers stress, directly impacting emotional wellbeing and resilience.

Public Health Equity:

Mobile units, insurance expansion, and education campaigns help underserved rural and semi-urban populations access quality dental care earlier, reducing health disparities.

By bridging the silence at an individual and systemic level, we do not just save teeth—we save time, costs, dignity, and opportunity.

Strategic Reflection

"Lessons Beyond Dentistry"

Conducting this research and engaging closely with patients taught me lessons that stretch far beyond the clinical realm. At its heart, this book is not only about oral healthcare delays—it is a study of human behavior, systemic inertia, and the pathways to sustainable change.

The key reflections that emerged from this journey are:

Behavioral Barriers Outweigh Awareness Gaps:

It is not always lack of knowledge that stops individuals from seeking care; it is fear, shame, mistrust, and procrastination. Solutions must therefore target emotions as much as information.

Trust is the First Treatment:

Building trust is not a soft skill—it is a strategic advantage. Whether in healthcare, consulting, or management, outcomes are dramatically better when stakeholders feel heard and respected.

Systemic Problems Require Cross-Functional Solutions:

True transformation never stems from one angle alone. Policy, technology, education, and community mobilization must work in tandem to achieve sustainable change—just as multi-pronged frameworks solve complex business challenges.

Inertia is Costly:

Just as delayed dental care leads to compounded health issues and costs, delayed organizational action leads to missed opportunities and declining performance. Recognizing inertia early is crucial to problem-solving.

Small Changes Drive Big Impact:

Even a few moments of empathetic conversation, a clear visual explanation, or a culturally sensitive campaign can shift behaviors dramatically over time. Change does not always need to be grand to be powerful.

Through this journey,
I learned that silence is not merely the absence of sound; it is the presence of unresolved fear, misunderstood behavior, and systemic friction.

Understanding silence—and bridging it—is not only critical for better healthcare, but also for better leadership, management, and change-making across industries.

Where Do We Go From Here?

The silence I studied wasn't just about pain.
It was about delay. Doubt. Dignity.

This book began as a research project. It became a listening exercise. Then a mirror.

What I saw in clinics, in camps, in waiting rooms—wasn't just dental anxiety.
It was people waiting for permission to care for themselves.

And in that space between neglect and need, I realized: we don't just need better healthcare.
We need better systems, better spaces, better stories.

We need policymakers who listen.
Clinicians who pause.
Families who ask.
Technology that softens.
Designs that invite.
And most of all—patients who believe that they matter.

This book offers frameworks, yes. But more importantly, it offers a call.

To every strategist, dentist, health worker, and leader reading this—
the silence will not break itself.

It will take policy that listens, clinics that heal, and communities that speak.

So where do we go from here?

We go forward—with care, with strategy, and with the courage to meet fear where it lives:
in the unsaid.

And then we begin—not just to treat,
but to transform.

EPILOGUE

This book began with questions. Quiet ones, almost too shy to speak aloud.

Why do people carry pain for months, even years, before seeking care?

But in the journey of writing, researching, and remembering, those questions transformed. They became more human, more layered:

What are they really afraid of? What kind of world do we need to create so they don't have to be afraid?

Through this work, I saw how clinical charts hold numbers, but not nuance. How check-up camps diagnose teeth, but not trauma. How behind every delay is not just procrastination, but a person longing to be understood without judgment—something my research clearly echoed when it showed that over 93% of participants delayed care, and the strongest reason was the belief that it wasn't necessary without symptoms.

I witnessed courage—not in the absence of fear, but in its presence. Patients who sat down despite trembling hands. Mothers who brought their children before themselves. Elderly men who whispered, "Pehli baar kisi ne poocha."

In them, I saw the power of presence. The healing that begins not with a drill, but with dignity. Not with expertise, but with empathy.

So if this book leaves you with anything, let it be this:

There is no such thing as a small act of care. Even a warm glance or a moment of stillness can feel like a bridge across fear. A hand gently resting on the armrest, a tone that says, "I see you"—these are not soft gestures. They are silent revolutions.

Whether you're a healthcare provider, a policymaker, a student, or simply someone with a heart—know that your tone, your patience, your softness can change the course of someone's journey.

We may not always cure.

But we can always comfort.

And that, too, is medicine.

Thank you for walking with me—through clinics and camps, through fear and silence, through facts and feelings.

Here, in the space between smiles, healing waits.

It waits in the pause before confession. In the courage to sit in the chair. In the softness that says, "Take your time."

Let's not rush it. Let's not ignore it. Let's stay.

FINAL NOTE

This book is more than a reflection of personal observation. It is a hybrid between:

Narrative Case Studies: Emotional experiences, raw patient dialogues, and real stories

Survey-Based Analytics: Quantified trends that reveal behavior patterns

Strategic Solutions Framework: Structured problem-identification and solution roadmaps

REFERENCES

1. American Dental Association (ADA). "The Psychology of Dental Fear."
2. Ministry of Health and Family Welfare, India. Oral Health Survey Reports.
3. Research questionnaire and data collected by Dr. Arushi Chandra, 2023-24 (unpublished).
4. Chandra, Arushi. "The Impact of Procrastination and Psychosocial Factors on Dental Attendance and Oral Health Status." Asian Journal of Dental Sciences, vol. 7, no. 1, 2024, pp. 387–396. https://doi.org/10.9734/ajds/2024/v7i1217.
5. Selected patient stories collected through observational fieldwork in 2023-24.
6. Sharma, R., et al. Pilot Study on Empathy Training and Patient Outcomes in Mumbai Dental Interns. Journal of Public Health Dentistry, 2021.
7. Corah, N. L. (1969). Development of a Dental Anxiety Scale. Journal of Dental Research, 48(4), 596.
8. Government of India. Ayushman Bharat Health and Wellness Centres: Operational Guidelines, Ministry of Health and Family Welfare, 2020.
9. World Health Organization (WHO). Oral Health Fact Sheet, 2022.

CALL TO ACTION

If this book touched you, moved you, or helped you see things differently, I would love to hear from you. Your feedback keeps these stories alive and helps them reach more hearts.

Leave a review on Amazon/Kindle

Share a favorite quote or chapter online and tag me

Connect with me on Instagram: @aaruuxxhiii_

Let's keep the conversation going—because silence only ends when we speak.

Thank you for being part of this journey.

The untold stories behind the silence.

In the everyday rhythm of Indian clinics and hospitals, much is left unsaid.
Bridging the Silence explores the unspoken truths of patient psychology, misunderstood intentions, and the systemic issues that influence care outcomes.

Written by a practicing dentist with a deep interest in public health, this book combines real-life observations with critical insight, helping both healthcare professionals and lay readers discover what truly happens when treatment meets human emotion.

Author's Bio

Dr. Arushi Chandra is a dental surgeon, researcher, and healthcare observer passionate about reforming patient experiences and provider understanding in the Indian medical landscape.

9 789334 285109

www.ingramcontent.com/pod-product-compliance
Ingram Content Group UK Ltd.
Pitfield, Milton Keynes, MK11 3LW, UK
UKHW021402190726
13845UKWH00028B/829

9 789334 285109